THE CHEMISTRY AND THERAPY OF BEHAVIOR DISORDERS IN CHILDREN

Publication Number 470

AMERICAN LECTURE SERIES®

A Monograph in

AMERICAN LECTURES IN LIVING CHEMISTRY

Edited by

I. NEWTON KUGELMASS, M.D., Ph.D., Sc.D.
Consultant to the Department of Health and Hospitals
New York City

THE CHEMISTRY AND THERAPY OF BEHAVIOR DISORDERS IN CHILDREN

By

HERBERT FREED, M.D.

Chief, Child Psychiatry Research Unit
Philadelphia General Hospital
Clinical Professor of Psychiatry
Temple University Medical School
Consultant in Psychiatry
Veterans Administration of Philadelphia
Philadelphia, Pennsylvania

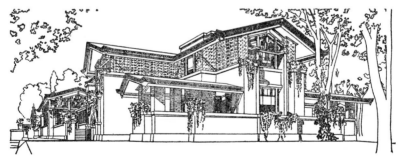

CHARLES C THOMAS · PUBLISHER
Springfield · Illinois · U.S.A.

CHARLES C THOMAS • PUBLISHER
BANNERSTONE HOUSE
301-327 East Lawrence Avenue, Springfield, Illinois, U.S.A.

© 1962, by CHARLES C THOMAS • PUBLISHER

Library of Congress Catalog Card Number: 61-17015

With THOMAS BOOKS careful attention is given to all details of manufacturing and design. It is the Publisher's desire to present books that are satisfactory as to their physical qualities and artistic possibilities and appropriate for their particular use. THOMAS BOOKS will be true to those laws of quality that assure a good name and good will.

Printed in the United States of America

FOREWORD

OUR LIVING CHEMISTRY SERIES was conceived by Editor and Publisher to advance the newer knowledge of chemical medicine in the cause of clinical practice. The interdependence of chemistry and medicine is so great that physicians are turning to chemistry, and chemists to medicine in order to understand the underlying basis of life processes in health and disease. Once chemical truths, proofs and convictions become sound foundations for clinical phenomena, key hybrid investigators clarify the bewildering panorama of biochemical progress for application in everyday practice, stimulation of experimental research and extension of postgraduate instruction. Each of our monographs thus unravels the chemical mechanisms and clinical management of many diseases that have remained relatively static in the minds of medical men for three thousand years. Our new Series is charged with the *nisus élan* of chemical wisdom, supreme in choice of international authors, optimal in standards of chemical scholarship, provocative in imagination for experimental research, comprehensive in discussions of scientific medicine, and authoritative in chemical perspectives of human disorders.

Dr. Freed of Philadelphia presents the cardinal principles of abnormal child behavior in terms of its prevention and treatment with psychotropic compounds. The term "behave" emerged in the sixteenth century to connote "have yourself" in hand to fulfill Nature's injunction: "be yourself!" Every organism seeks to be master of its own fate within the limits of time, chance, and circumstance. The insurgent quality of life with its capacity for initiating unexpected activities to overcome its inner limitations and outer handicaps is as characteristic as the more tangible attribute of motility. But growth, development, and training of self-regulation, self-direction, and self-discipline enable the child to live up to arbitrary standards of behavior set for his chronological age, intellectual achievements, and social adjustments. The author interprets the problem child not only as a symptom of problem development but of problem environment in health and disease with all the clinical implications of chemical therapy. It helps bring the organism and the environment into mutual harmony, partly by modifying the organism to fit the environment, and partly by modifying the environment to fit the organism. The slow rate of establishing such an equilibrial system by psychologic and psychiatric procedures may now be accelerated by the newer chemical compounds that react with deep-seated brain centers, i.e., tranquilizers, hallucinogens, central stimulants. This newer psychopharmacology emerged from paleolithic pharmocology. Ecclesiasticus XXXVIII, 4 c. 180 B.C. teaches us "The most High hath created medicines out of the earth, and a wise man will not abhor them." The return to Aesculapius in quest of mental health attests to the development of child psychiatry in terms of clinical chemistry, for all nervous mechanisms produce their effects through the intermediary of chemical substances. *In animo perturbato, sicut in corpore, sanitas esse non potest.*

I. NEWTON KUGELMASS, M.D., PH.D., SC.D., *Editor*

PREFACE

I⊤ WOULD SEEM to be a common practice in psychiatry to set a five year interval after the advent of a new therapeutic approach as the minimal period of observation essential for an objective evaluation of the results of that therapy. Since it is more than five years since reports on the "tranquilizers" for the emotional disturbances began to appear, this fact could be given as the justification for this publication. However, there are other perhaps more vital motives. Though the use of drugs for the emotional disturbances of children is not new since Bradley (30) popularized the use of the amphetamines, psychopharmacotherapy has just crossed the threshold of global therapy with whole families of new and potent drugs. One cannot summarily dismiss the host of favorable reports on these drugs for varied conditions in adults or the smaller group of studies on emotionally disturbed and mentally handicapped children.

The major drive for this survey is the urge to work toward a possible union of psychopharmacology and psychodynamic psychiatry. The child guidance clinic ushered in the widespread recognition that in treating a child we are really treating the family unit rather than a single patient—the child. Today we are entering the era of family treatment and analytic family therapy with further acceptance of the family as a unit. Simultaneously we are being deluged with literature on a variety of drugs which can profoundly modify behavior through direct effects on the central nervous system.

With full awareness that many pediatrists and psychiatrists are opposed to the use of tranquilizers for children or have issued cautions such as "most reports are limited to initial clinical impressions" (50), this survey will attempt to evaluate the present status.

vii

CONTENTS

THE CHEMISTRY
AND THERAPY OF
BEHAVIOR DISORDERS
IN CHILDREN

Chapter I

PSYCHOPHARMACOLOGY AND/OR PSYCHODYNAMIC THERAPY

BASIC TO THE DISCUSSION of the psychopharmacologic actions of the tranquilizers and the antidepressant drugs are the formulations of Hess (78) for which he was awarded the Nobel prize in 1949. He regarded the diencephalon rather than the cortex as the "true control organ of the body," and located the central tracts in the diencephalon and the mesencephalon which correlated the activity of the sympathetic and parasympathetic nervous system and higher brain functions. The functional integration of the diencephalon with the extrapyramidal motor system is called the "diencephalic motor innervation." He called the central representation of the sympathetic nervous system the ergotropic system and the central representation of the parasympathetic system the trophotropic system. These two systems act reciprocally, contributing to the regulation of behavior ranging from apathy and sleep following electrical stimulation of the trophotropic system to excitement and mania with stimulation of the ergotropic system. Brodie (38) who had reported that reserpine discharged serotonin and norepinephrine from the brain speculated that norepinephrine could be a synaptic transmitter for the ergotropic system and serotonin a transmitter for the trophotropic system. Brodie utilized these observations to theorize about the action of reserpine as a tranquilizer after his series of studies showed that reserpine discharged both serotonin and norepinephrine from the brain and also from binding sites elsewhere in the body. It is vital to note that only those analogs of reserpine that lowered the brain amine content produced sedation. Furthermore the sedation appeared to result from the fact that unbound serotonin continued to be formed at nerve terminals at a rate faster than its local inactivation and also to be in excess of the discharged norepineprine. It was concluded that the serotonin thus spilled over at its synaptic junctions stimulating the trophotropic division of the Central Nervous System (C.N.S.) (37). Brodie further proposed that an excess of serotonin would be tranquilizing whereas an increase of noradrenaline is stimulating.

Neurophysiologists and workers in psychopharmacology have isolated four important functional areas of the brain. These are the reticular formation, the limbic system, the hypothalamus and the cortex. The function of the cortex and the influence of drugs on it is well known compared to the observations listed for the other areas. The hypothalamus is the location from which all of the autonomic functions mentioned above are regulated. The limbic system or visceral brain consists of the hippocampus, the amygdala, the fornix and the olfactory cortex. Animal experiments indicate a close relationship between the limbic system and the emotions. The reticular arousal system comprises the reticular formation in the brain stem and the midbrain. It controls wakefulness and sleep. It is claimed that the varied clinical effects of the tranquilizers can be correlated with differing neurophysiological effects on these functional areas of the brain, e.g., the phenothiazines do not affect the cortex but do stimulate the hypothalamus while the reticular formation is slightly depressed. In contrast, the propanediols such as meprobamate do not affect either the cortex or the hypothalamus but do depress the limbic system and may slightly stimulate the reticular formation (24). The amygdala (amygdaloid nucleus) is found to respond to both chlorpromazine and reserpine with abnormally increased neurophysiologic activity. Thus we have to realize that while one part of the brain involved in emotional responsiveness is hyperactive there can be a simultaneous depression of function by release of hormones such as adrenaline, noradrenaline and serotonin which are parts of the mobilization mechanism, e.g., the fight-flight response of Cannon. Berger (24) has suggested that the low reactivity of the hypothalamus in many psychotic patients could be responsible for schizophrenic symptoms by producing a type of sensory deprivation and thus evoke symptoms such as hallucinations. It would follow that drugs which would stimulate the hypothalamus could be therapeutic to psychotic patients.

Saunders (143) has proposed that psychoses are a disorder of the regulation of metabolic processes rather than an insufficiency of certain enzymes or of essential neurohumoral metabolites. An example of a dynamic amine equilibrium is the histamine-catechol-amine (e.g., epinephrine) relationship. The tranquilizers which inhibit transamination and the hydrazines which inhibit deamina-tion probably act through chelate formation of the pyridine, flavin or porphyrin catalysts. The synthesis of the more potent phenothia-zines has suggested to Ayd (8) that the clinical effects of each drug can be attributed to a selective affinity for different subcortical areas. The increased incidence of extrapyramidal symptoms is correlated with greater activity in the limbic system where the amygdaloid nucleus and the hippocampus are particularly involved. In contrast the weaker phenothiazines exert their greatest depres-sing effect on the hypothalamus and on parts of the reticular system.

Attempts have been made toward the ultimate integration of psychopharmacology and psychodynamics. Ostow and Kline (128) have used the psychoanalytic structural concepts of the psyche: ego, superego and id and discussed the distribution and utilization of psychic energy in this system. I have found this unconvincing as have some other analysts. A substantial formulation with a more firmly based neurophysiological foundation is that of Lehmann (112). He noted that neurophysiologic research has demonstrated differences in synaptic transmission in the various structures of the central nervous system with the result that the same psychopharmacologic agent may facilitate transmission in one system and inhibit it in another. He then postulates three func-tional organizations in the central nervous system: (a) the viscero-psychic system composed of the "visceral brain" in the limbic lobe, the reticular activating system and the autonomic nervous system. It deals primarily with the awareness of affects in its orientation;

(b) the sensoripsychic system which depends on more highly structured stimuli transmitted by the long sensory pathways to the cortex. This system is object-conscious or reality-conscious in its orientation; (c) the cortico-psychic system which is maintained by internuncial stimuli and it chiefly shows concept-conscious or symbol-awareness in its orientation. He concludes with the proposition that excessive activity of any of these systems, whether absolute or relative within this balance may result in severe disturbance of the ego and therefore will be manifested as psychiatric illness. Lehmann has found that many of the tranquilizers are characterized by ability to inhibit visceropsychic responses strongly while interfering only slightly with the more vulnerable sensoripsychic and corticopsychic functions. Thus they bring about a favorable change of balance in the pathologically deranged equilibrium of the ego. The strength of the ego depends on the relative strength of the corticopsychic and sensoripsychic systems as compared with the visceropsychic system. This visceropsychic system is looked upon as the most primitive system and thus less vulnerable to noxious agents. In sensory deprivation, a state widely investigated and discussed these days, it is suggested that a relative excess of visceropsychic and/or corticopsychic activity results.

Some workers in psychopharmacology such as Irwin (94) are convinced that the differences in behavior between higher animals and man are more quantitative than qualitative. He is convinced that the "behavior profile of a drug" can be more thoroughly evaluated in animals than in man and that on the basis of this profile, within limits, one can predict the potential value of a new drug in the treatment of mental disease. The suppression of conditioned avoidance behavior and of locomotor activity are major behavioral responses to the phenothiazines in humans and animals. Further development of the training of animals so that we can selectively develop and measure behavior patterns tied in with various emotions is now being achieved. (36, 121). Others like DiMascio and Klerman (52) believe that the bridges between animal work and human studies are as few as the bridges between the findings in normal humans and patients.

Irwin (93) has also suggested that the similarities between the behavior of animals and humans should make one consider the use of drugs to produce a "therapeutic community." He has shown that by treating the most disruptive individuals of groups of animals one may be able to provide an atmosphere of social harmony conductive to the development of more social attitudes and behavior. Besides giving many references on the control of aggressive-destructive behavior, anxiety and resistance to handling of animals he is also impressed by the possible pertinence of imprinting.

Imprinting has been considered as an extremely rapid form of learning. It is differentiated from instinctive behavior by the ethologists in that it takes place only during a very brief critical period of the organism's life. While it has been studied chiefly in birds, Huxley (92) suggests that human beings are subject to what he calls "a peculiar form of imprinting known as romantic love," taking place around puberty. He reminds us that imprinting on songbirds does not take place until they are a year old or coming into maturity.

The pertinent significance of imprinting for us in the cortex of psychopharmacology lies in the observations of Hess (79) on the imprinting of mallards. The imprinting period was extended by the use of meprobamate or chlorpromazine. The anxiety formerly shown to strangers was eliminated at the termination of the critical imprinting period. We can only keep in mind the distant possibility that such observations may have pertinence to the learning problems (e.g. reading) of young humans.

To utilize the psychopharmacologic approach most effectively, requires to my mind, a dynamic approach to psychotherapy. We can outline this with four major points:

(I) MAKE EMOTIONAL CONTACT

While this is a "must" in the dynamic approach to any patient, it is especially so with children since they are usually brought unwillingly to the doctor. They do not come as patients but have to be converted from what might be called an unwilling fellow traveler into a patient. Play therapy usually paves the way toward emotional contact. Perhaps this need to make the contact with the child a moving one is most vividly expressed in existential psychiatry. One speaks of the "encounter" between the patient and the doctor with the therapist exhibiting "presence." The intangible union which should follow is vital for it fosters the wish to be understood. Often early resistance is shown by institutionalized children who fantasy that taking medication indicates that they are "crazy." Their deeper feelings of isolation and rejection become more pervasive. We have observed that the feeling of being accepted stressed by Bender as an effect of the amphetamines with some children also seems to develop in some of the seriously regressed youngsters following the exhibition of stelazine.

(II) CULTIVATE AND MODULATE THE AFFECTS

The technique of encouraging abreaction popularized by David Levy in child psychiatry made a place for itself but now child analysis has modified the emphasis on affective release. When we realize that every learning experience is an affective experience we can appreciate the importance of cultivating the affects. Kierkegaard stressed that anxiety could be our greatest teacher. This is encompassed in Freud's formulation that small quantities of anxiety (signal anxiety) facilitate the readiness for adaptation. For many patients, however, a greater degree of anxiety is disorganizing and does not aid the learning process. Today we are frequently able to modulate the affects of fear, shame, and aggression with the tranquilizers (see discussion of reading disability, etc.).

The young child has been labeled "motor minded" since he expresses his vitality in action and in the non-verbal expression of affects. The tempo of the action dialogue of youth can often be slowed with selected drugs to the pace which leads to understanding rather than chaos. In the older child and adolescent we appreciate by contrast that verbalization must be looked upon in many cases as useful only as the carrier for affect. We are indeed fortunate that the sense of wonder and the feeling of enthusiasm so often lacking in adulthood can be cultivated in childhood. Perhaps the current research on reward and punishment systems in the brain by Lilly (114) will one day be complemented by psychopharmacologic studies leading to greater specificity and localization of effect on the brain.

(III) FOSTER INTROJECTION

The psychoanalytic concept of introjection was pictured clearly and simply by the little boy who said, "When I am close to you, I do not feel alone inside."

The pill often becomes a transference symbol. The placebo effect is only a minor facet in the utilization of this process of introjection or identification. The learning process can be looked upon as a process of incorporation or introjection. The old school master intuitively knew this when he taught the alphabet and reading with the aid of the ingestion of alphabet soup. The current emphasis on the development of ego identity suggests to us that this quest for identity may become even more important than the search for insight. Existential psychiatry points that way also in focusing upon the "encounter;" so does the psychoanalyst when he displays increasing willingness to be a "real person" to his patient. The child psychiatrist cannot evade this function.

(IV) CONVERT THE INTERPERSONAL COMMUNICATION INTO THE "DIALOGUE WITH ONESELF"

This is the ultimate goal of therapy. Of course it is accented more in adult therapy than in child guidance where psychic structures are in a state of flux and the mother-child relationship is undergoing a subtle disengagement. The therapist and the patient seek to learn each other's emotional language. We will fail the child as he builds his perceptual world if we do not help him to see it clearly. But it is in the gradual development of this ability to stand off and see the self thus finding that "psychic distance" which makes each of us realize we are never really alone inside. Psychic distance is needed for insight. This initiates the dialogue with oneself.

When we emphasize that the therapist and the patient seek to learn each other's emotional language we are implying also that there must be a clarification of the transference- countertransference relationship. This relationship in child therapy differs from that in adult therapy since the child is still relating intensely (on a non-symbolic level) to his parents while the therapist in his relationship to both the child and his parents also alters the usual counter-transference relationship. The use of the pill may strengthen oral dependency strivings and further fixation at this level. This potential for regressive behavior is often held up by those therapists who postulate a basic incompatibility exists between psychotherapy and the giving of drugs (145). Savage makes the comparison, "It is the difference between giving food and giving food for thought."

Obviously I am in disagreement with the conviction that psychopharmacotherapy and psychotherapy for children are incompatible. The relative infrequence of the combined approach of drugs and psychotherapy in the child guidance clinic stems from many factors. Besides justified caution about unproven approaches there is an admitted lack of knowledge about such agents because of therapeutic complacency. An exaggeration of such complacency is the countertransference attitude that if one should need to add drugs as adjuncts to verbal therapy that therapist has suffered a narcissistic trauma. As a masterful adult he has been unable to deal with a disturbed child. A related countertransference problem is seen in the therapist who is unconsciously determined that he will "always be in control of" the treatment relationship even if he has to subdue the patient with tranquilizers. And of course the unconscious determination to "get the patient well" may also lead to the same undesirable countertransference response.

The symbolic significance of the administration of a drug as either a hostile, a sexual gesture or a magical gesture are familiar concepts intimately related to the topics of transference and placebo effects.

Essentially then, the transference-countertransference relationship in the child psychiatry clinic is more complex than that seen in the adult clinic and resolution of the transference is not a goal of treatment. But an understanding of the transference-countertransference situation especially modified by the additional variable, the drug, is vital in achieving the maximum benefit from treatment.

BOX I

The beneficial effects of chlorpromazine (Thorazine), reserpine (Serpasil), triflupromazine (Vesprin), prochlorperazine (Compazine), trifluoperazine (Stelazine), meprobamate (Equanil, Miltown), hydroxyzine (Atarax, Vistaril) for children with emotional disturbances have been studied now for from two to over five years. The therapeutic effects in both children and adults would seem to be ameliorative rather than curative. (It must be emphasized that the evaluation of a drug in the growing child is different from that in the adult where the processes of maturation play a minor role.) Today, the symptomatic approach with the use of the psychopharmaceuticals as an adjunct to psychotherapy can be advocated for selected cases. It is recommended that the therapist acquire a background of experience with just a few drugs rather than continually experiment with newer drugs as they appear. In this way he will be able to recommend an effective dosage more quickly and be more completely informed about side effects. He must constantly keep in mind that while each of the potent drugs can be said to have a psychopharmacological profile the reaction of the child patient to the medication will be the resultant of the many factors involved in the therapeutic situation.

Chapter II

TRANQUILIZER THERAPY

T ODAY, ONE CAN say with confidence that the newer psychopharmacologic agents which would include both the tranquilizers and
the anti-depressants, have an established place in the treatment of
the emotional disturbances of adults (4, 87). Hoch, a pioneer in
this field, specified further that more attention must be paid to
integrated treatment, drugs and psychotherapy, by experts in the
field of psychotherapy. Can such observations be made in the field
of child psychiatry? One must admit upon surveying this field that
it is in a state of flux (84).

A report by Fisher (61b) on Child Research in Psychopharmacology shows that more reports with better research design are needed
to validate the initial favorable papers just as the relatively small
number of reports on children treated intensively with child
analysis calls for more studies and workers in this field when compared to those reports from the child guidance clinics. Certainly
the child analytic studies are lighting our way toward a better
nosological classification just as they are leading our children toward better mental health. The analogous potentiality that our
knowledge of the psychodynamics and the neurophysiology of the
growing child may be expanded by the exhibition of psychopharmaceuticals to the child is not sufficient justification for their use.
The best interests of the child does necessitate the maximal recognition of his right for self-determination, growth and the working
out of conflicts (155). But we must accept the existence of the
active interest of the public and of our profession in seeking the
quicker way to mental health. If we agree that truth is a direction
and not a destination let us see if this may be a way.

The scope of this monograph will be limited to a clinical discussion of those psychopharmacological agents which are listed as tranquilizers and the central nervous system stimulants which include the new anti-depressive agents which have been reported to be useful in child psychiatry. Only those drugs are listed which have been utilized in child psychiatry by the author or other workers. It will not include the barbiturate or non-barbiturate sedatives or the anti-convulsive agents.

Following the suggestion of Schiele and Benson (146) we have divided the tranquilizers into the major agents which include the phenothiazine derivatives and the rauwolfia derivatives, and the minor agents which include the substituted propanediol derivatives, meprobamate and phenaglycodol (Ultran) as well as the diphenylmethane derivatives such as hydroxyzine (Atarax) (99).

MAJOR TRANQUILIZERS

a. Phenothiazine Group

Chemical Name	Generic Name	Trade Name	Average Daily Dose
2-chloro-10-(3-dimethylaminopropyl) phenothiazine	Chlorpromazine	Thorazine	30-150 mgm
10-(3-dimethylaminopropyl) phenothiazine	Promazine	Sparine	30-200 mgm
2-chloro-10-[3-(1 methyl-4-piperazinyl) propyl] phenothiazine	Prochlorperazine	Compazine	10-30 mgm
2-chloro-10-[3-(1-B-hydroxyethyl-4-piperazinyl)-propyl] phenothiazine	Perphenazine	Trilafon	2-6 mgm
10-(3-dimethylaminopropyl)-2-trifluoromethylphenothiazine	Triflupromazine	Vesprin	20-50 mgm
10-[3-(1 methyl-4-piperazinyl)-propyl]-2-trifluoromethylphenothiazine	Trifluoperazine	Stelazine	1-6 mgm
10-[3-(1-B-hydroxyethyl-4-piperazinyl)-propyl]-2-(trifluoromethyl) phenothiazine	Fluphenazine	Prolixin	.25-1.5 mgm
2-methylmercapto-10- 2-(1-methyl-2-piperidyl)-ethyl phenothiazine	Thioridazine	Mellaril	20-75 mgm

b. Rauwolfia Group

Chemical Name	Generic Name	Trade Name	Average Daily Dose
Trimethoxybenzoyl reserpate	Reserpine	Serpasil	.5-3 mgm

MAJOR TRANQUILIZERS

It has been proposed that the primary action of the phenothiazine compounds is to depress the physiologic accompaniments of the emotional factors of the personality. The affective state which results can be looked upon as a modulated fight-flight response (Cannon) in that the aggressive patient is calmed while the withdrawn patient may show productive or "normalized" behavior (82). Of course, this description of the drug effect on the central nervous system is oversimplified. The psychologist Skinner (150) pointed out that in humans "avoidance behavior" may take such forms as flight, immobility, aggression, repression, compulsions, delusions and possibly even hallucinations. The test for avoidance behavior as carried out in animals may seem to be quite removed from those human behavioral manifestations listed above. The experimental technique requires the use of a conditioned stimulus, e.g., a buzzer in conjunction with an unconditioned stimulus, generally a noxious and punishing one such as an electric shock. During a training period the animals learn to avoid being shocked by moving into a defined safety area such as climbing a pole or in case they do not avoid, to escape from the shock into a safety area. During conditioning trials the animals learn to respond to the buzzer. When this recurs regularly a conditioned response has been developed when the animal does not jump at a stimulus but does jump from shock while under the drug influence there has been a suppression of the conditioned avoidance escape response.

When we talk about the specific effects of a number of therapeutic agents, it is implied that we can expect the response of the patient to be predictable depending on the known action of the drug. This may be far from the fact. Indeed, in dynamic psychiatry, the formulation that it is not the traumatic event but the meaning of the event to the patient which determines the seriousness of the trauma applies equally well in explaining drug effects. A detailed analysis shows that beside the test agent and its mode of administration, the nature of the symptom to be treated, the motivation of the patient and the physician, as well as the life situation of the patient at the time of treatment determine the reaction of the child to the drug. Furthermore, with children we must go beyond this because the child alone cannot be considered as the therapeutic unit responding to the potent agent. The unit is even more than the child and the parents for in some cases the teacher must be included. Indeed, in many of our cases the social worker, or sister from a religious order attached to a residential institution and in close contact with the patient, can be seen to respond vigorously to changes in the child. The mechanism of circular causality or the "feed back phenomenon" is obviously involved. Certainly then, the response to the drug in the growing organism can encompass a broad spectrum of reactions. With this perspective, statements about the unpredictability of action or the transient beneficial effects of psychopharmacologic drugs occasionally seen in the emotional disturbances of children may be better evaluated.

CHLORPROMAZINE

A comparison of the clinical effects of the various members of the phenothiazine group has led to efforts to divide this family into two or three model groups. One model is chlorpromazine, another is prochlorperazine and there is a small group which can be labeled miscellaneous (see Chapter I). A drug in this group would be Mellaril. The members of the prochlorperazine group are much more likely to produce basal ganglia dysfunction. Their dose range is therefore restricted.

We reported on the use of chlorpromazine for hyperkinetic emotionally disturbed children in 1956 (68). The twenty-five patients served as their own controls. Improvement was noted in over 80% of the patients who were treated for periods ranging from four to sixteen months. Eighteen of the patients were classified as primary behavior disorders. While the most prominent change was a lessening of over-activity and the basic character make-up remained the same, the faculty for learning seemed improved in 20% of the cases. In five of the patients enuresis was decreased. Contact was maintained with the majority of these patients during the intervening years with the aim of determining the possibility of harm to their personality development.

Since our observations on these children, who did not require hospitalization, there have been at least three (73, 91, 123) of 46 or more children, each in residential centers. All reported a beneficial response in the areas of hyperactivity and aggressiveness. Schizophrenic children tended to improve also. Possibly the most significant study was that by Freedman *et al.* (71) in thirty-two children. This was well designed. The statistical conclusion was drawn that chlorpromazine was particularly useful in the treatment of hyperkinetic children, principally in those whose hyperkinesis was associated with schizophrenia. Fish (59, 60) has summarized her satisfactory experiences in the adjunctive use of drugs in the private practice of child psychiatry since 1952. Chlorpromazine was one of the phenothiazines found useful.

Since some of our school children showed an improvement in learning while taking the chlorpromazine for disturbed behavior we undertook another study on four matched groups of boys who had reading disabilities (69). The use of reading instruction combined with chlorpromazine was found to be superior to that of reading instruction alone and to be superior to the results obtained when chlorpromazine alone was used. The best results statistically were obtained with the combined use of reading instruction and chlorpromazine. These results suggested that there was an added advantage to the use of this combination over reading instruction alone. The combined use of prochlorperazine and reading instruction was also found useful, with a trend that approached statistical significance. The clinical observations in the small group so treated suggested that the adjuvant use of prochlorperazine was probably even more promising than that of chlorpromazine. No disturbing side effects were noted with either drug. This study convinced us that in view of the extent of reading retardation and the possibility that such retardation is an index of psychopathology the use of the selected tranquilizer as an adjuvant to reading instruction seems worthy of trial. The limited availability and costliness of reading instruction makes any such adjunct worthy of investigation.

In the five year interval following the initiation of adjunctive therapy with chlorpromazine we have followed fifty-two patients for periods varying from two to over four years and a greater number for the same interval who have been taking prochlorperazine. The children did not seem to develop a tolerance to the drugs although about one out of five taking the chlorpromazine (average dose 25 mgm t.i.d.) and one out of eight taking the prochlorperazine (average dose 10 mgm b.i.d.) complained of occasional drowsiness during the school period in the first month of treatment. Subsequently such complaints were infrequent. We cannot refrain from observing that their teachers rarely complained. Indeed it is likely that in many cases they were grateful as these catalysers of class room tension were removed.

The parents were informed that the medication was to be stopped immediately if the child developed a sore throat or if a rash developed. Two patients developed skin eruptions which subsided with withdrawal of the drug. Another drug was substituted without untoward effect.

Irwin (93, 94) has reported that tolerance develops rapidly to the suppression of avoidance behavior but very slowly or not at all to the suppression of locomotor activity in the test animals. We have the impression that an analgous response was seen in the children with primary and secondary behavior disorders where the major complaint (of the parents and teachers) was hyperactivity and not the subjective complaints of anxiety, phobias, etc.

These children were given a battery of psychological tests which included Wechsler Bellevue, Rorschach, Bender Gestalt, "Draw a person" test as well as specialized tests when indicated. The changes in personality dynamics were not dramatic, but improved facility in reading and mathematics occurred to a degree which could be described as a trend approaching statistical significance $(P < .05)$.

Finally a comment on the technique for termination of treatment. We tried to have the drug withdrawn gradually to prevent a possible resurgence of symptoms. However, we found that the unplanned for sudden termination of treatment did not produce a predictable return of symptomatology. It was therefore concluded that withdrawal symptoms did not occur.

PROCHLORPERAZINE AND TRIFLUPROMAZINE

To date we have utilized prochlorperazine (Compazine) in more than one hundred patients. The availability of the spansule form as well as the usual tablet which thus makes the one dose form practical for the school child accounts in part for the larger population given this drug. We have also used trifluopromazine (Vesprin) (64) in thirty children from this same clinic population over a thirty month period of observation. The range of diagnoses covered the entire nosological spectrum of childhood with the majority of cases classified as primary behavior disorders. Our current impression is that either of these drugs will be as effective as Thorazine. In addition there is a diminished incidence of drowsiness in doses comparable in clinical effectiveness such as 20 mgms of compazine per twenty-four hours or 30 mgm of Vesprin per twenty-four hours instead of the usual 25 mgm of Thorazine t.i.d.

However, one side effect of Compazine was noted in two of the patients receiving 15 mgm. spansules b.i.d. which was disturbing to the child, the parent and to the doctor. It was the development of dystonic involvements of the head and neck. These manifestations are more commonly seen in adults receiving larger doses of the drug and usually have been classified with the better known evidences of Parkinsonism which appear relatively frequently when the more potent phenothiazine derivatives like Trilafon, Prolixin and Stelazine, as well as Compazine, are used. In the past few years at least ten reports (16, 44, 46, 76, 77, 96, 120, 127, 147, 149) have appeared in which alarmed parents and even doctors have rushed children to the hospital who had taken these drugs (in most cases Compazine) for nausea and vomiting and had then reacted with such disturbing side effects. The child was usually thought to have some C.N.S. disease and spinal punctures were performed. Even heroic measures like tracheotomy were tentatively considered because of the localized spasms of musculature. In view of our relatively extensive experience with Compazine as well as Prolixin and Stelazine in children and adults we feel that this side effect is dramatic but not dangerous and is not as frequent as one might gather from reading the above mentioned reports. It can be avoided in almost every patient if the initial dose of the drug is small and the effective dose is approached gradually. Only the rare idiosyncratic case will react undesirably. By making the parental figure and the referring doctor knowledgeable the occurrence will no longer provoke a crisis. A final point (66) can be made that the use of an anti-Parkinsonian agent and antispasmodic such as cogentin or Benadryl given intravenously or intramuscularly as a specific corrective practically always results in a recovery which is just as dramatic as the onset of the symptoms have been. Finally, it must be clarified here that while we have suggested that Compazine and Vesprin are comparable in action we have not come upon this type of extrapyramidal side effect following the recommended dose of vesprin in children.

Mention must be made here of a report (50) which is a model for research in the out-patient clinic in which prochlorperazine and meprobamate were used as the potent tranquilizers and compared with the effect of the placebo. The placebo effect was found to be equivalent to that of each of the other drugs. It is significant that twenty-two of these children were subsequently placed on perphenazine and there was a definite trend in favor of perphenazine. The authors highlighted the fact that the diagnosis rather than the drug correlated with the favorable outcome. Thus the "neurotic" children showed substantial improvement while the "hyperkinetic" children showed moderate gains and a group of defective children with behavior disorders and an anti-social group showed a negligible response.

STELAZINE

A trifluoromethyl phenothiazine, trifluoperazine (Stelazine) which has been found effective in adult psychotics was studied by us for its efficacy in markedly disturbed children. Although there is a series of reports on adults the paucity of such with larger populations of sick children treated in an out-patient clinic (67) induced us to report this data in some detail. A series of twenty-three children ranging in age from two to seventeen years was given Stelazine in doses ranging from 2 mgm to 20 mgm daily.

Seven children were classified as schizophrenic (childhood), two as autistic children and the remainder as severe behavior disorders. All of the patients received the drug from six to fourteen months except two who took it for three and four months respectively.

The children in this study came from foster homes or institutional placements. Because psychopathology abounded, only superficial supportive therapy was given in addition to the psychopharmacologic agents. The efficacy of the Stelazine was highlighted in that fair to excellent results were obtained in fifteen patients and thirteen of these had failed to respond satisfactorily to other tranquilizers. The latter included prochlorperazine, chlorpromazine, meprobamate and phenaglycodol. Two patients with childhood schizophrenia and one with an autistic state were among those responding with excellent results.

Eight of the patients manifested side effects which necessitated the stoppage of the drug. These effects were typically manifestations of the basal ganglia dysfunction such as dyskinesic movements involving the head and neck and rarely the Parkinsonian symptoms of oculogyric crises, fixed facies and restlessness (akathisia). All of these findings disappeared when the drug was stopped. While it had been our experience that the size of the dose does bear a direct relationship to the incidence of such neurologic dysfunctions as it does in adults (7), there can also be an idiosyncratic reaction in some patients to smaller dosages which occurs repeatedly on fresh trials. Many of these patients thus react unfavorable early in the course of treatment (7). One can then usually assure the parental figure after the initial observation period of a few months that the patient will stabilize on that particular dose and not require such closely scheduled evaluations. It is significant that some of the patients were found to have cerebral dysrythmia in their EEG tracings but the use of stelazine did not produce seizures in any of these patients nor did the subsequent EEG patterns suggest further dysfunction.

An example of an excellent response is the case of P. R., a female first seen at the clinic in 1955 when she was five years old. The complaint was that the patient was having staring spells, seemingly unaware of her surroundings, was aggressive and hyperactive, even being restless in her sleep. She was also destructive, unfriendly and unaffectionate. While she ate well she had to be fed. She was in a foster home and did get considerable care and attention from her foster parents but the child could relate to no one. She would knock her head against the floor or wall, smiled inappropriately, made faces to herself and was completely oblivious to her surroundings.

Psychologic examination at that time showed the patient to be retarded. The electroencephalogram was definitely abnormal with a persistently fast brain pattern. The abnormal high voltage, slow frequency waves and sharp waves were considered indicative of a cortical dysrhythmia. She was diagnosed as having an organic behavior disorder with associated cortical dysrhythmia. In view of her cerebral dysrhythmia she was first placed on phenobarbital and sodium dilantin and continued on this from 1955 until July, 1956. At this time because she did not improve and because of her marked aggressiveness and destructiveness, she was placed on chlorpromazine 10 mgm three times a day along with phenobarbital $\frac{1}{4}$ gr. three times a day. The patient showed no improvement on this medication and in August, 1956 the phenobarbital was discontinued but the chlorpromazine 10 mgm three times a day was continued. She was rechecked at monthly intervals with little or no improvement. In December, 1956 it was reported that she was a little quieter and that she had learned bladder control but generally speaking had not shown marked improvement. Finally, in September, 1957 the chlorpromazine was stopped and she was placed on phenaglycodol. She still was described as a fearful, restless, inattentive, destructive child. She was now definitely autistic and was considered to be a case of schizophrenia when reviewed by the clinic staff. As of November, 1957 she was sleeping better but showed no other change in her conduct. She remained without medication from November, 1958 until January, 1959 at which time she was placed on Stelazine, 2 mgm. four times a day. Showing improvement from the initiation of this phase of treatment she was maintained on 2 mgm. of Stelazine four times a day. She was re-examined psychologically in July, 1959 and the psychologist reported she was no longer hyperkinetic in that while she was active the activity was not aimless. She was now very talkative and she could be understood although her speech was indistinct. She tried very hard to repeat words. She was more friendly, was playing more with the other children, was enjoying automobile trips and was very affectionate with everyone in the family, particularly the male adults. She improved to the extent that she was able to attend school and joined in the class activities enthusiastically. She made clay models and trays and was very affectionate to the other children though very shy. While she still seemed to go into trance-like states, an escape into fantasy, she was more in contact with reality and during the summer months was able to go to the seashore. She lost her phobia for water, became more meticulous about herself and also enjoyed her own swimming pool in the backyard. She enjoyed picnics and parties and was obedient. On her examination on December 10, 1959 her foster mother painted a remarkable picture showing that a complete change had taken place in the past year with the patient. She had been taking Stelazine 2 mgm four times a day and now had lost much of her fear and anxiety, and all her phobias. She was not destructive; in fact her foster mother brought in toys she had been playing with in the past year that were not even scratched. She played with them continually and she preserves them very carefully at present. She was now curious, she sat with the examiner asking questions and listening to replies quietly and obediently. She was friendly and affectionate and accepted any demonstration of attention without fear and anxiety.

At this time, the child is definitely considered a schizoid child and is emerging from a severe autistic state after several years of medication. The response to stelazine was considered remarkable. She is now taking Stelazine 2 mgm four times a day.

The value of Stelazine in the seriously disturbed child with normal intelligence has been confirmed in a smaller group of children by Fish, and in two larger groups of mental retardates (see section on mental deficiency).

While it may be premature to theorize on the explanation for the greater effectiveness of Stelazine for the psychotic or seriously disturbed child, a review of the literature does offer clues. Mac-Donald *et al.* (118) have observed that Stelazine effectively eliminated or modified aggression and hostility. This action has also been attributed to Thorazine. The uniqueness of Stelazine may lie in the cliam made for it by Kovitz (103). He believes that Stelazine acts both as an ataractic agent to calm aggressive patients and as a stimulant to stir passive, sluggish patients into productivity and contact. A clinical observation of great importance confirmed by a number of workers is the tendency of delusions and hallucinations to drop away in response to stelazine therapy. Lehmann and Knight (113) have given eighteen healthy volunteer subjects their battery of psychophysiologic tests in conjunction with the administration of Stelazine. The results imply that the drug acts selectively to decrease perceptual intake and psychomotor speed and at the same time to increase attention, concentration and general vigilance, thus increasing the ability to handle this input. If one recalls that agents such as mescaline which can produce psychotic states has the effect of increasing sensory input we find a possible psychophysiologic explanation for the antipsychotic action of Stelazine.

PROLIXIN

Prolixin which ranks Stelazine in being one of the most potent of the phenothiazines has been given to eighteen children with primary behavior disorders. The average dose was 1.5 mgm in twenty-four hours and the top dose was 3 mgm per twenty-four hours. Moderate to excellent improvement was noted in twelve of the cases observed over an eight month period. It was concluded that this preparation probably exhibited the same advantages and disadvantages of the preparation Stelazine on which we are making an extended report in this article. However, it must be emphasized that a patient population of psychotic children similar to those treated with Stelazine was not available for the exhibition of Prolixin.

PROMAZINE

Promazine (Sparine) has been exhibited to mental retardates (see mental deficiency). It has also been combined with meprobamate as Prozine (53) and given to 193 difficult management problems in a custodial institution. The effective daily dose was 600 mgm of meprobamate and 75 mgm of promazine. The authors found that the synergistic action of the combination succeeded where the single ataractic agents had been ineffective. The fact that the doses of promazine in relation to body weight are greater than they are for chlorpromazine or most other phenothiazines and thus makes for a greater likelihood of the side effect of convulsions, makes this a minor drawback in the use of this drug.

THIORIDAZINE

Thioridazine (Mellaril) is now under investigation in our clinic since it has been reported to have therapeutic efficacy in adults with an absence of extra pyramidal side effects, convulsions and other less serious complaints. Our preliminary study on less than twenty patients with primary behavior disorders in doses of 30 to 50 mgm daily has been encouraging. Observations with a period of observation from six to twelve months thus far do confirm the absence of side effects other than drowsiness. A favorable report on the treatment of 21 children diagnosed as having an organic hyperkinetic behavior syndrome was made by Zarling and Hogan (163). Increased attention span was found in 79% of cases, a decrease in classroom blowups in 71% of cases, and control of hyperactivity in 63%. An enlightening table (47) on some of the phenothiazines in the treatment of adults is in agreement with our observations. In March, 1961, Pauig *et al.* (132) reported that Mellaril was not only an aid in the control of behavior disorders of the institutionalized epileptic but also in the reduction of epileptic seizures.

RESERPINE

There are few reports on the use of reserpine on emotionally disturbed children (not mentally defective) compared to the large number of studies in which the drug was tried on adults. That of Zimmerman (164) is an excellent study in which 130 children were treated for a minimum of six months. It was found that 75% of the experimental group of children and adolescents showed improve-

IMPORTANT SIDE EFFECTS AND COMPLICATIONS WITH COMMONLY*
USED PHENOTHIAZINE DERIVATIVES

Compound		Complication or Side Effects					Extrapyramidal Syndromes		
Generic Name	Commercial Name	Blood	Liver	Epileptic Seizures	Skin	B.P. Fall	Parkin- sonisms	Dys- tonias	Aka- thisia
chlorpromazine	Thorazine	+++	+++	++	++	++	++	+	+
mepazine	Pacatal	+++	++	-	-	-	-	-	-
perphenazine	Trilafon	-	-	+	+	+	+++	+++	+++
prochlorperazine	Compazine	+	++	+	+	+	+++	+++	+++
promazine	Sparine	+++	++	+++	+	+++	++	+	+
promethazine	Phenergan	-	-	-	-	-	-	-	-
thiopropazate	Dartal	-	-	-	-	-	++	++	++
thioridazine	Mellaril	-	-	-	-	-	-	-	-
trifluoperazine	Stelazine	-	-	+	-	+	+++	+++	+++
triflupromazine	Vesprin	+	-	+	-	++	++	++	++

Legend +++ = major problem; ++ = occurs often; + = rarely seen; − = not reported

*Cole, J. O.: Drug Therapy. In-Spiegel, E. A. (Editor): PROGRESS IN NEUROLOGY AND PSYCHIATRY (Vol. XV, 1960), Grune & Stratton, New York, 1960 (by permission).

ment compared to improvement in less than 40% of the control group. The findings from a battery of psychological tests showed that the verbal, motor and social intelligence test ratings improved slightly in both the control group and the "reserpine" group. But the Rorschach testing found there was an improvement in the quality of control in one-third of the patients as compared to one-seventh of the controls. The inference might be drawn from this battery of test material that motor and affective responses were significantly influenced while ideation was not. Experimentation with dosage led to an average dose of 1.5 mgm daily; drowsiness was the major side effect and was controllable with dose modification. It should be noted that Kline (100) has recently emphasized that the period of observation with therapy employing reserpine must not be less than six months. This was carried out in the above study.

The other interesting report is by Lehman *et al.* (111) in which doses up to 5 mgm daily were given to nine autistic children with beneficial results in all. They were surprised to find an exacerbation of psychotic symptoms when the drug was withdrawn. There was definite evidence that both the awareness of others and relatedness improved during treatment. Our own results with reserpine were not as impressive as those seen with the phenothiazines. The action was rather unpredictable in our experience as it was in that of Bender and Nichtern (23). We must admit that we did not persist in using the reserpine for a six month treatment period as Kline now recommends. This could account for the unimpressive results (101) .

MINOR TRANQUILIZERS
MEPROBAMATE

Meprobamate is said to influence the subcortical areas which comprise the "Papez circuit" (the thalamus, cingulate gyrus and amygdalate nucleus) , without affecting the reticular activating fibers. This Papez circuit which integrates the crude awareness of the older cerebral parts with the discriminative aspects of consciousness arising from cerebral cortical activity is rendered less sensitive by barbiturates. They relieve muscle spasm by decreasing conduc-

MINOR TRANQUILIZERS

A. Alkanediol Type (Propanediol)

Chemical Name	Generic Name	Trade Name	Average Daily Dose
2-methyl-2-n-propyl-1, 3-propanediol dicarbamate	Meprobamate	Miltown Equanil	400-800 mgm
2-p-chlorophenyl-3-methyl-2,3-butanediol	Phenaglycodol	Ultran	300-600 mgm

B. Diphenylmethane Type

1-(p-chlorobenzhydryl)-4-2-(2-hydroxyethoxy)-ethyl piperazine	Hydroxyzine	Atarax Vistaril	20-50 mgm
2 (Benzohydryloxy)-N, N-dimethyl-ethyl amine hydrochloride	Diphenhydramine	Benadryl	30-150 mgm

tively along long internuncial pathways. They raise the convulsive threshold to electrical and chemical stimulation and do not affect conditioned reflexes. From the psychological viewpoint meprobamate can be said to raise the frustration threshold.

It is probably to be expected that there would be a number of papers on the use of meprobamate in the emotional disorders of children since such emphasis has been put on its low toxicity and the relative freedom from side effects. It has therefore been given to infants as an ideal anti-tesion drug as well as to children from age two. The many manifestations of tension such as irritability, restlessness, poor eating and sleeping patterns, night mares, head banging, tics as well as enuresis, stuttering, nail biting and reading disability are all reported to have responded favorably (11, 23, 70, 98, 104, 116, 122). The trend toward favorable reports in modifying many aspects of psychic dysfunction is matched by the reported failures of the drug to significantly modify the psychotic states, particularly childhood schizophrenia (104, 134). There are no convincing favorable reports on the value of meprobamate in serious delinquency. Our findings in the treatment of symptoms such as irritability, restlessness, nightmares and other sleep pattern disturbances is likewise favorable just as our observations confirm the failures of others to induce remissions in childhood psychosis.

Meprobamate has been found to be the most useful of a group of tranquilizers which can act as adjunct in treating irritability, restlessness, apprehension and sleeplessness in handicapped children. Many of these children had cerebral palsy and the mental development of some is within the limits of normal. Baird (11) reported on a large series (210 patients) of such children ranging in age from two months to fourteen years in which he used the long-acting form (Meprospan) where the contents of the capsule could be mixed with the food. Improvement resulted in 109 of the 210 children and the possibility of side effects was minimized by the extended dosage form. This is a practical consideration in the treatment of children attending school, etc., where the single dose form is desirable. The symptomatic improvement made the family more enthusiastic about working out a therapeutic routine which held the promise of emotional growth. It was found that the effective dose was between 25 and 60 mgm per kilogram per day for the child with cerebral palsy, while the other patients did not need more than 10 to 15 mgm per kilogram per day. Katz (97) studied nineteen children in a cerebral palsy school and found that nine of ten children when given an adequate dose of meprobamate (enough to adequately control muscle spasm and involuntary movements) completed the school year with an increased attention span and an improved ability to learn. This lead to a better assimilation of information and faster school progress.

Among Baird's patients were fourteen classified as children with "brain injury." Following the lead of Strauss (154) he thus categorized children with marked distractibility, short attention span and erratic behavior although they did not have a history suggesting a previous encephalitis. Only four of these children (29%) responded favorably. In contrast Carter (41) claimed that the behavior problems of brain-damaged patients—both children and adults—"almost vanished" in 57% of cases and were markedly or moderately relieved in 97% of forty-seven patients given meprobamate.

The "hyperkinetic syndrome in epileptic children" (129) characterized by the same cluster of symptoms: hyperirritability, hyperactivity, belligerence and short attention span, is more of a problem to parents and teachers alike than convulsive seizures which are relatively infrequent. A report (117) on 128 epileptic children of whom 59% also manifested hyperactive behavior disorders indicated that the behavior difficulties were alleviated. On the other hand, although meprobamate has anticonvulsant properties (5, 12, 90, 134) Livingston's patients with major motor, petit mal or psychomotor seizures were not significantly relieved. Only minor motor seizures were influenced favorably in some cases. While other types of seizures may be increased the lack of toxicity makes the drug indicated where the emotional overlay is important, in our opinion.

By this time there are enough reports on the possibility of habituation to meprobamate and the withdrawal effect that comments must be made on two recent significant reports. Hollister (88) has been investigating tranquilizer reactions for years. Before the American Federation for Clinical Research he reported that meprobamate withdrawal effects are related to dosage levels. Using a double blind study he found that only ten out of sixty adults who were on moderate therapeutic doses had withdrawal symptoms but that sixteen out of twenty-one who had been on extremely high dosage (4.8 gm to 8 gm) developed tremors, insomnia, emotional lability and gastrointestinal distress. Withdrawal symptoms appeared within twenty-four to ninety-six hours after the drug has been replaced by placebo (89). A similar type of double blind study was made on forty children, age ten to sixteen years, with varied diagnoses. Improvement was noted in 65% of the patients. We would emphasize the observation that abrupt withdrawal of meprobamate caused a temporary sharp increase in tension, agitation and anxiety. Convulsions were observed in two children in whom a latent convulsive tendency subsequently was confirmed by E.E.G. recordings (138).

HYDROXYZINE

Hydroxyzine (Atarax) (Vistaril) is another minor tranquilizer which was found useful in child psychiatry since 1955 (6-80). With an average dose of 30 mgm. daily in divided doses side effects were rare and not serious. The minor behavioral disorders where hyperactivity was characteristic responded best. Bayart (17) in an extensive report on 187 children ranging between one and twelve years of age reported that most of over forty children suffering with tics responded favorably within two weeks and in 78% of the cases, the recovery was complete. Not having had personal experience with this preparation, we can only say that such a favorable and prompt response in the treatment of tics as well as the other positive reports make this drug worthy of consideration for specialized indications. A recent report (115) claims control of 93% of the presenting symptoms in forty-one patients which included quarrelsomeness, insomnia, hyperactivity, school phobia, facial tics and anxiety.

STIMULANTS AND ANTI-DEPRESSANTS

Chemical Name	Generic Name	Trade Name	Average Daily Dose
dl-1-phenyl-2-amino-propane sulfate	Amphetamine sulfate	Benzedrine	5-30 mgm
d-2-amino-1-phenylpropane	Dextro-amphetamine	Dexedrine	5-15 mgm
2-dimethylaminoethyl 4-acetylaminobenzoate	Deanol	Deaner	100-150 mgm
1-isonicotinyl-2-isopropylhydrazine	Iproniazid	Marsilid	Not recommended for children
B-phenylisopropylhydrazine	Pheniprazine	Catron	Drug withdrawn
B-phenylethylhydrazine	Phenelzine	Nardil	5-30 mgm
Methyl-a-phenyl-2-piperidineacetate	Methylphenidate	Ritalin	30-80 mgm
5-(3-dimethylaminopropyl)-10, 11-dihydro-5H-dibenz-[b,f]-azepine	Imipramine	Tofranil	10 mgm b.i.d.
5-(3-dimethylamino-propylidine)-dibenzo [a,d] [1,4] cycloheptadiene hydrochloride	Amitriptyline	Elavil	10 mgm b.i.d.

DIPHENHYDRAMINE

A. Freedman (70) who pioneered in the use of drugs for the behavior disorders in children with Bender, introduced the use of diphenhydramine (benadryl) for the primary behavior disorders and disturbing habit patterns, prior to the advent of the tranquilizers. He still finds it useful to control impulsive behavior in doses of 30 to 150 mgm daily. Fish (59, 60) made the interesting observation that the efficacy of the drug in diminishing anxiety is markedly diminished when the child is over ten years old. She postulates that it has "an organizing effect on immature motor incordination and impulsivity."

Chapter III

STIMULANT THERAPY

IN COMPARISON TO the tranquilizers, the stimulants are few in the psychomotor stimulants, such as the amphetamines. In addition to the amphetamines which have long been recommended for the control of behavioral problems for children we now have new number but increasing as psychic energizers (101) are added to agents comprising part of the group of the anti-depressants toward which so much attention is directed today. It is significant that while the syndrome of depression is uncommon in children (140) these drugs have been found useful in the treatment of various aspects of emotional disturbances in children.

The AMPHETAMINES (amphetamine and dextro-amphetamine) have been used for the control of behavior problems in children since Bradley first reported on their use in 1937. His interest in this area is evidenced by a series of reports (30, 31, 32, 33, 34, 35). He found that withdrawn, lethargic children tended to become more alert with an increasing show of happiness in social participation while aggressive, hyperactive children tended to become less quarrelsome and calmer. Laufer (109), an active worker in the field of psychopharmacology for children has found dextro-amphetamine superior to chlorpromazine in a group of disturbed children. He demonstrated that a diagnostic procedure (a low threshold to metrazol stimulation) could be used to delimit this group which he considered to be an organic behavioral syndrome. The common symptoms are hyperactivity, poor powers of concentration, irritability, impulsiveness and explosiveness. Laufer found that the administration of amphetamine sulfate raised the threshold to that of the normally healthy group.

The observations over the past twenty years which include reports by Bender (22) and Hill (81) make it apparent that the amphetamines have an established place in the treatment of hyperactive and aggressive behavior patterns in children. It has been suggested by Hill that tolerance to the amphetamines may be used as a clinical diagnostic test for the aggressive behavior pattern in children. He has found that they may tolerate daily doses of 60 mgm of amphetamine sulphate without disturbing their sleep pattern. A major indication for the exhibition of the amphetamines is the treatment of enuresis where we may see the same type of tolerance to larger doses. Hodge (86) has outlined a treatment of dosage of amphetamines for enuresis. He suggests the initial dose of 5 mgm of Benzedrine (d-l-amphetamine) on going to bed. The dose can be raised to 20 or 30 mgm daily depending upon the change in the enuretic pattern or the appearance of insomnia or anorexia. The dose of Dexedrine (d-amphetamine) is about one-half that of Benzedrine. It should be noted that the data from several reports suggests that the results with Benzedrine were superior to those with Dexedrine. Both Bender and Freedman found these drugs ineffective in the treatment of psychopathic and schizophrenic children (22, 70) .

It has been suggested by Hodge (86) that the amphetamines alert the cerebral cortex through the reticular activating system. It is interesting that the clinical observations on the effect of the amphetamines suggest that they tend to "normalize the behavior" of disturbed children in that they make the aggressive overactive child quieter and the withdrawn child more active socially. This effect is similar to that of the potent tranquilizers on child behavior in that they appear to modulate the fight-flight response. The tranquilizers are now considered the classical drugs which influence the reticular activating system.

The MONAMINE OXIDASE INHIBITORS are the potent stimulants in current favor and there are a few reports on their use in children. The term psychic energizer has been applied to this group in contrast to the amphetamines which are called stimulants (144) . The behavioral effects induced by these monamine oxidase inhibitors are in marked contrast to the stimulation by an amphetamine in their intensity and time course, i.e., immediacy of effect and cumulative effect. It is significant that amphetamine elicits obvious hyperactivity immediately after injection while the MAO inhibitors often cause depression after injection. The rise in brain serotonin concentration after MAO inhibitor administration is used as a screening test for potential antidepressants in the laboratory. It is presumed that these inhibitors act as energizers by stockpiling enough free norepinephrine to stimulate the ergotropic division.

Hoffer (85) notes all of the energizer drugs are related to the catecholamines. He adds imipramine to the sympathomimetic amines, e.g., amphetamine and methylphenidate with a structure similar to adrenaline. In a related group he puts iproniazid and the MAO inhibitors and thirdly he suggests that imipramine may be in the group with cocaine in that they sensitize adrenergic synapses.

Freedman (70) stated in a preliminary report on iproniazid (Marsilid) in the treatment of fourteen autistic children that seven were definitely improved so that the early results were considered promising. A dose of .5 to 1 mgm per pound daily over a six month period was given. Marsilid was found to be an effective but toxic drug in adults and also in children so that a number of safer effective monamine oxidase inhibitors are now available. One of these is phenelzine (Nardil) which was used in a three year study of a group of twenty-nine children from six to twelve years of age and 68 children from the age of twelve to sixteen years suffering, apparently, with behavior disorders. These patients were institutionalized and the observations made during their school attendance indicated that they were more attentive and cooperative although their academic achievement remained poor (143).

After emphasizing the difficulty of making a diagnosis of the psychiatric entities in childhood, Saunders went on to say that "Phenelzine in a majority of children resulted in a relaxed cooperative individual with less aberrant responses to emotional stimuli, relief from sexual drives and improved relationship with their associates." The dosage of phenelzine (Nardil) was 15 mgm b.i.d.

initially and adjusted up to 15 mgm t.i.d. depending on the clinical response. The maintenance dose level was 5 mgm. Sleeplessness was a disturbing side effect in approximately 8% of the patients. The other report (135) on the use of this same family of drugs in children utilized Catron, chemically (1-methyl-2-phenyl) -ethylhydrozine hydrochloride, a cogener of amphetamine. Perlstein (135) exhibited it to 123 children with diagnoses of cerebral palsy, epilepsy and emotional and behavioral disturbances. Substantial benefit was noted only in the seventy children with various types of behavioral disturbances. Improvement generally consisted of a diminution of irritability and hyperactivity. The patients generally had a longer attention span and seemed more in contact. The side effect, sleeplessness, occurred in over 20% of the cases. Catron has been withdrawn from the market because of some visual disturbances observed after the administration of higher dosages to adults. This action emphasizes that caution must be exercised in using a member of this family of drugs. It also highlights the fact that a particular drug may be very closely related chemically to another effective and safe drug, i.e., amphetamine, but not be safe itself thereby necessitating a period of observation before using these potent agents in the growing organism.

Deaner (deanol) (2-dimethylamionethyl 4-acetylaminobenzoate) is a precursor of choline and thus to acetylcholine. It has been used by Oettinger (125). He reported favorably on the responses of 108 non-epileptic children who had responded poorly to at least one other agent including the amphetamines, chlorpromazine and rauwolfia derivatives. Most of the children manifested behavioral problems and were diagnosed as belonging to the group characterized as "brain injured." The average dose was 50 mgm given daily in the morning. Most of the patients were observed for periods of from nine to fifteen months. Improvement occurred in 68%. Seventeen epileptic children were also treated and seven of these became more disturbed so he concluded that the amphetamines were the preferred drugs for this group. Oettinger felt that deanol offered the advantage over the amphetamines in improving behavior without inducing "jitteriness," anorexia or insomnia. At present he is recommending higher dosages (about 150 mgm) (126). Palmer and Wright (131) reported that Deaner increased attention span, educability and the happiness of eight retarded children. However, the best controlled study (45) evaluated the changes occurring in two matched groups of twenty retardates using doses up to 150 mgm for an eight week period. From the elaborate test battery findings it was concluded that the few suggestive changes could be assumed from a tranquilizing effect of Deaner, rather than a specific improvement in concentration or span of attention. In the latest study (74) it was felt that puzzle solving ability and organization of ability improved after a ten week period of 100 mgm daily in children diagnosed as having behavior disorders. The findings were not impressive. Our findings in an uncontrolled pilot study soon after the advent of the drug were likewise unimpressive other than the freedom from side effects. We did not attain the 150 mgm dosage.

Methylphenidate (Ritalin) Methyl a-phenyl-a-2-piperidylacetate is another stimulant and analeptic. It differs from amphetamine in lacking adrenergic action. Knobel (102) reported beneficial responses in fifteen of twenty children who were classified as having behavior disorders associated with organic brain disease. The period of observation varied from one to eighteen weeks with the dose ranging from 80 to 100 mgm daily. He believes that pathophysiological effects in the cortex are favorably influenced by the methylphenidate. The stimulant effect overcomes the maturational lag which underlies the behavioral disturbances. Another paper (51) dealing with the same category of children also used methylphenidate. However no data was given of the dose, number of cases treated or the outcome.

With the success of imipramine (Tofranil) 5- (3-dimethylaminopropyl) -10, 11-dihydro-5H-dibenz- [b,f] -azepine, as the first of a new family of antidepressants, this drug has also been recommended for emotional disturbances in children (adolescents) . However, depression as a specific entity is rare in children and the indications, specific or non-specific, have not as yet been adequately reported. Another member of this same family, amitriptyline

(Elavil) has also been found effective in a spectrum of cases in adults that extends beyond the various types of depressions to include the anxiety states (63). Amitriptyline (Elavil) is 5-(3-dimethylamino-propylidine) - dibenzo [a,d] [1,4] cycloheptadiene hydrochloride. In imipramine, the central seven membered is azepine, the nitrogen replacing the partially unsaturated carbon of the amitriptyline cycloheptadiene ring. Because the side effects were minimal and the drug has a tranquilizing quality, being closely related to chlorpromazine, it is now being used in our clinic for selected cases. To date only ten children (six with primary behavior disorders, two with reading disability and two with behavior disorder secondary to organic brain disease) have been given the medication in doses of 10 mgm. t.i.d. and observed for periods extending from one to three months. The response was fair to excellent in all but three cases.

BOX II—MENTAL DEFICIENCY

There is evidence that various phenothiazines are effective in improving the adjustments of a significant number of disturbed mentally deficient children. Side effects may occur more frequently in the lower grade retardates and thus interfere with the efficacy of the drug. There is no conclusive evidence indicated that educability is promoted by the exhibition of the tranquilizers. It is possible that the utilization of the tranquilizing effect to promote psychotherapy and perhaps facilitate a positive transference relation may further the process of reeducation. This is an important goal of all forms of therapy.

Chapter IV

CLINICAL CITATIONS
MENTAL DEFICIENCY

In 1956 KUGELMASS published his observations on the psycho-chemotherapy of mental deficiency in children (105). He observed that "the heterogeneity of presenting problems veered this study toward single symptoms or specific manifestations in all types of amentia for this five year study." Even though this excellent survey reviews the comparative effectiveness of ten widely used psycho-chemotherapeutic agents for a variety of symptoms, only one pheno-thiazine, chlorpromazine, is included. This suggests the extent to which we are being deluged with new preparations, and the pheno-thiazines are now in the vanguard (1, 3, 14, 15, 18, 22, 26, 27, 40, 49, 62, 64, 65, 68, 71, 73, 75). Bair (10) compared the effects of chlor-promazine on ten hyperactive mental defectives with ten untreated children matched in age, sex and I.Q. There was an average in-crease of 10.4 points in the I.Q.s of the drug treated group as com-pared to an increase of 2.5 points in the untreated group. Behavior-al improvement also occurred. Essen (57) subsequently reported the same trend in two similar comparative groups. These and other papers (139) also confirmed the value of chlorpromazine for the control of psychomotor excitement in the mentally deficient.

When reserpine was the tranquilizing medication and a con-trolled double-blind study was carried out with 130 high-grade retarded children no significant difference was found between the drug and placebo groups (141). In the latest report by the same group (142) Compazine (prochlorperazine) was used as the tran-quilizing agent. Contrary to expectations and the reports of pre-vious observers (29, 48, 124) the gains made by the compazine subjects were generally less than those evidenced by the group which received placebos and the third group which took nothing. The superiority of the placebo subjects over the control as well as the drug subjects suggested that a "placebo effect was as effective, if not more so than the actual chemical therapeutic action of compazine." In a similar fashion the favorable reports on Reserpine by Fisher (61), Timberlake *et al.* (159) and Pallester *et al.* (130) can be opposed by Rosenblum *et al.* (141, 142) and Wardell *et al* (161). Disturbed behavior was the major indication for the treatment of many groups and there are favorable reports on the effects of chlorpromazine by Tarjan *et al.* (157), Bair and Herold (10), Essen (57) and Rettig (139) while Ison (95) found no significant changes in the intellectual level. Craft (48) utilized a number of drugs and applied a statistical analysis to the rating scales. He concluded that Compazine was superior to chlorpromazine to a statistical degree in controlling hyperactive behavior. He also found that side effects seemed more frequent in the lower grade retardates.

Anothr phenothiazine, promazine (Sparine) has been effective (20, 56). Benda reported on seventy six patients treated over a ten month period with moderate improvement seen in fifty three patients. It was pointed out that chlorpromazine had been given previously without appreciable benefit. A milder tranquilizer with minimal side effects, hydroxyzine (Atarax), was utilized in a study of sixteen matched pairs of educationally subnormal and maladjusted children. Improvement in both behavior and performance in fourteen out of sixteen patients was noted while only two taking the placebo responded.

The studies in which Himwich (83) participated offered the broadest spectrum of treatment utilizing the most potent phenothiazines. The patients were disturbed retardates ranging in intelligence from idiot to high grade moron and in age from nineteen to forty seven. In 1958, chlorpromazine was found superior to reserpine and promazine. In 1960 triflupromazine (Vesprin) and trifluoperazine (Stelazine) in doses of 100 to 300 mgm were efficacious but significant side effects were present in about 10% of the patients. It must be noted that convulsions did not occur although these had occurred in some of these same patients when they were given one of the group or reserpine, thorazine, pacatal or sparine previously.

Tarjan's report on research in mental deficiency (156) gives us a useful orientation for discussing any therapy with tranquilizers. He pointed out that intelligence in general is influenced by an infinite number of variables and therefore the distribution of intelligence should be demonstrable according to the Gaussian distribution curve. However, the actual number of mental defectives is found to be in excess of the theoretically expected figure. Tarjan is convinced that this finding and others suggests that the deficient population can be mentally divisible into two basic categories: the so-called "physiological" and the "pathological" groups. The excess group would encompass the "pathological group." The physiological category outnumbers the other by a ratio of approximately 16 to 1. Patients in this group are generally mildly deficient, blending gradually into the continuum of the general population. Most of the patients in the physiological group come from a below average socio-cultural background. Cultural stimulation, intellectual curiosity and scholastic endeavors are not highly valued by the families. Enrollment in school, adolescence, sexual maturation, job finding are good examples of the stress periods which demonstrate the emotional vulnerability of the physiological group. In the pathological groups of mental deficiencies the I.Q. is likely to be below 50 with concomitant somatic signs and brain histopathology. The diagnosis can be suspected and made early. Tarjan (156) finds that superimposed neurotic and psychotic manifestations occur more often and are precipitated by a lesser degree of stress than that required to make "normal" children ill.

There are two studies on the effect of trifluoperazine on the training of mentally defective children. Carter speaks with five years of experience in this area with both the major and minor tranquilizers (42) . Trifluoperazine was exhibited to forty one emotionally disturbed mentally defective children who had responded poorly to the other medications. With an average dose of 10 to 15 mgm daily the majority of the patients became more sociable and productive in addition to developing an improved appetite and sleep pattern. He concluded with the conviction that "trifluoperazine is a potent agent that can produce benefits where other drugs have not."

The second report (110) was also favorable and brought out that behavioral symptoms marked by violence appeared to be the most responsive to therapy very early in treatment. Within six months of using doses up to 8 mgm daily, training had produced marked improvement in the eating habits of all the higher-grade and autistic children and marked improvement in the habits of nine of the eighteen imbeciles. Thus thirty seven had good to excellent results. Extrapyramidal side effects were minimal and easily controllable

BOX III—BEHAVIOR DISORDERS

Both the major and the minor tranquilizer as well as some of the stimulant drugs have been found useful in the behavior disorders of children with and without brain damage. But wherever possible, the drug therapy should be an adjunct to some form of psychotherapy. Drugs should be used only in an attempt to prevent personality disorganization rather than to abolish anxiety. The patient with the typical picture of neurosis as seen in the adult should not be given tranquilizers except as a last resort.

BEHAVIOR DISORDERS—THE MILDER EMOTIONAL DISTURBANCES OF CHILDHOOD

The behavior disorders of children are probably a most important indication for the use of tranquilizers today. This is the large category which can be further subdivided into primary (with a psychogenic basis) and secondary (where organic factors are considered responsible for the deviant behavior.) This diagnostic grouping is distinguished from the neurotic disturbances where the clinical picture approaches the picture of neurosis as seen in the adult and from the psychotic states. The necessity to institutionalize some of these patients with behavior disorders as well as the need to treat behavioral manifestations in school children which would otherwise produce group disorganization had given us a major indication for the use of the tranquilizers (major and minor) as well as the amphetamines. As the efforts to delimit groups of these children by finding pathophysiologic bases for their aberrant behavior increase the category of primary behavior disorder grows smaller. It would seem that the reluctance to administer the newer drugs to the aforementioned group largely exists because of the conviction that such an approach will not resolve the primary disturbed interpersonal relationships of the family. But the adage—there are no problem children, only problem parents—the banner cry of the child guidance clinic, is not as hallowed these days. The studies of Mahler (119) on the symbiotic type of childhood schizophrenia and that of Escalona (25, 55) on constitutional factors, like the perceptive capacities of emotionally disturbed children, suggest that we may have under-emphasized the importance of constitution in the genesis of psychopathology in problem children.

The many tranquilizers and the amphetamines have been reported to be effective in both types of the behavior disorders. The anticonvulsant action of meprobamate along with the absence of Parkinsonian effects may give this drug a priority in some patients with behavior disorders with an organic basis. Laufer (108) has found the amphetamines superior to the phenothiazine chlorpromazine in behavior disorders presumably related to a pathophysiologic disturbance.

A number of symptoms associated with the behavior disorders, disturbing habit patterns, such as temper tantrums, head banging, enuresis, tics, stuttering, nail biting, have responded favorably although not consistently to both the major and minor tranquilizers. We have found that the entity "school phobia" which can be classified as a behavior disorder or as a childhood neurosis depending upon the extent to which associated fears are present can sometimes respond dramatically to the use of the more potent tranquilizers. An understanding of the psychodynamics of the particular patient is useful in explaining the alternation of symptoms and their prognostic importance.

Bradley (32) who pioneered in child psychiatry by introducing the use of the amphetamines now suggests that we can use the tranquilizing drugs for psychiatric emergencies. These would include the anxieties aroused when facing hospitalization, an operation or other of life's crises. He is convinced that the danger of dependency on these drugs is very slight because of the well known reluctance of children to take medicine.

For clinical pictures similar to the neuroses in adults, such as phobias and obsessive compulsive states where the child himself complains, medication is the last choice. It can be indicated if the level of anxiety threatened to produce a serious disorganization of the personality and psychotherapy is not available in any form. Delinquent behavior of varying degrees is often manifested by children classified as having behavior disorders. It has been our experience that while the tranquilizer can diminish tension and modulate the agression which may underlie sociopathic behavior the drug usually "does not give me a conscience" as one patient put it.

THE PSYCHOSES
(THE SEVERE EMOTIONAL DISTURBANCES)

This group includes autistic and symbiotic states as well as the typical picture of childhood schizophrenia. Positive results with the use of reserpine, chlorpromazine, prochlorperazine and triflupromazine, are reported but there is a possibility that trifluoperazine is the most effective agent currently available. Fish (60) agrees with us (67) on the values of trifluoperazine. She also reported favorably on perphenazine (Trilafon). At the risk of being repetitious, it should be noted that meprobamate was not found useful in this group of children.

BOX IV—LEARNING DISORDERS

The relationship between emotional conflict and impaired learning is unquestioned. There is not yet conclusive evidence that psychopharmaceuticals will improve the learning process in children with either normal or subnormal intelligence. But there is suggestive evidence that the adjunctive use of chlorpromazine, prochlorperazine, trifluopromazine, trifluperazine and meprobamate can modulate the affects contributing to emotional conflict. Such therapy can be considered in the global approach toward helping the slow learner and the child with reading disability.

LEARNING DISORDERS—SLOW LEARNERS AND READING DISABILITY

Children who are not achieving intellectually in school can be divided into two general groups: (a) the mentally defective and (b) those who are not mentally defective and are for a variety of reasons under par pupils. These are the slow learners, Dr. A. H. Wetter, superintendent of Philadelphia's public schools stated (28) that about one-third of the school enrollments were culturally handicapped by slow learners. This appraisal of the slow learners is generally accepted for each of the fourteen largest U. S. cities. A recent study made by school officials of the background of 117 slow learners and forty five average pupils in four high schools revealed that only 11% of the slow learners possessed adequate economic standards, a stable family, responsive parents and freedom from emotional disturbances. If one accepts the definition of psychic trauma as an experience which interferes with the learning process the psychological aspects of this problem become apparent. Coming from the environment they do, these slow learners cause massive behavior problems in the school. Reading becomes a major obstacle for the slow learners. Some have incredibly short memory spans— so short that they look at very familar words as if seeing them for the first time.

Our experience over the last five years suggests that remedial reading is a significant therapeutic adjuvant although progress is most likely to occur when psychotherapy and remedial reading are combined. Teachers have reported to us that the adjuvant use of the tranquilizers such as prochlorperazine, trifluopromazine, and more recently thioridazine in the lower dose levels, thereby diminishing tension, has helped the slow learners. The effect on class moral, the unconscious response of the teacher as well as the specific reaction of the medicated child probably complemented each other.

A dramatic result is worth a comment here. A twelve-year-old girl of superior intelligence was referred to us because of a reading disability and the inability to realize her full potentialities. This child had been examined in a highly regarded child psychiatry clinic when she was in the second grade of school. The mother was told about the daughter's reading disability which included the typical letter and word reversals. The mother then reported her frequent observations that the girl preferred to look at television while lying down in such a way that such an observer could only see a picture upside down. A thorough check up in the guidance clinic as well as the opthamology clinic showed that she perceived words reversed and rotated upside down. Following a complete workup the parent was told that the case was most interesting but not susceptible to a psychological approach since significant emotional conflict in the child and in the family constellation was not elicited. Nothing more was done by the mother in the years that followed until she was told by school authorities to contact us since we had started a research project on reading disability. We pointed out that we could not include the girl in the project, which required matched groups, since we had many boys with the handicaps and not enough girls. We offered her a possible palliative, prochlorperazine, as an immediate form of therapy and tentatively remedial reading and psychotherapy at an indefinite future date. The mother was very skeptical about the possible benefit of medication but accepted it when she was assured it could do no harm even if it did not help.

The patient was given prochlorperazine 10 mgm b.i.d. To her amazement and our own she returned with the child after a week of therapy, reporting that the child's ability to read had been helped markedly both in her own opinion and that of the teacher. Reading reversals became rare. On placebo medication there was a return of the difficulties. In subsequent interviews with the patient the feelings of shame and fear were highlighted as affects which had been present and were now removed as the child felt more like the other children. She had succeeded in hiding her difficulty before by the intensive use of her memory. The relationship between perception and emotional disturbances (58, 133) is highlighted by this case but cannot be discussed here except to note that a tranquilizer like prochlorperazine may produce a psychological and psychophysiological influence that would be beneficial here (151) .

We were impressed with the efficacy of prochlorperazine, Compazine, in the children who received it in the research project on reading disability (67). The clinical impression of all of the observers seemed to corroborate Lehmann's psychophysiologic test findings of increased attention and general vigilance in the healthy volunteer subjects to whom prochlorperazine was administered. We were also impressed by the pithy observations of Dr. Lauretta Bender (21) who stated, "Some of our follow-up studies have been completed in several hundred schizophrenic and non-schizophrenic children. From a therapeutic point of view, what we learned was that there was no therapeutic program that could materially or statistically change the course of a child's life. On the positive side, there is evidence that if problem children have a reading disability regardless of other diagnosis or factors and receive adequate remedial reading tutoring they improve in every respect." Another observer (104) used meprobamate to remove reading disability and was able to report positive results while we have been experimenting with triflupromazine, trifluoperazine, fluphenazine and thioridazine for reading disability.

BOX V—SIDE EFFECTS

It would seem that children are less prone than adults to develop side effects with the potent tranquilizers. Agranulocytosis has never been reported in patients under eighteen years old. Jaundice and severe dermatitis apparently are also quite rare in this same age group. The common side effect is drowsiness, readily controlled by lowering the dosage. The most dramatic but not the most dangerous side effect is basal ganglia dysfunction which may be idiosyncratic. Removal of the drug or lowering of dosage will remove the symptom. The placebo effect occurs just as frequently in children as it does in adults.

Chapter V

SIDE EFFECTS

SIDE EFFECTS OF drugs are a greater concern to the therapist when treating the child than when he treats the adult because the psychopharmacologic approach is an elective in treating children. It is therefore most reassuring to report that in our experience we have not seen a serious complication such as agranulocytosis, jaundice or a serious dermatitis in any of our cases. In the four cases from over 300 studied where skin eruptions were reported the condition cleared up when the drug was stopped. Two cases could be proved to relate to the use of chlorpromazine and one to the use of prochlorperazine. The rash was maculo-erythematous and confined to the trunk. It is also reassuring to learn from the A.M.A. Committee (2) which collects reports on agranulocytosis associated with drug intoxication that there is no report of a patient of age eighteen or under who developed agranulocytosis after taking a phenothiazine. Indeed, Hollister (88) collected the reported cases and found that most of them occurred in women over the age of fifty years. A search of the files of S.K.F. (152) for reports on cases of jaundice and severe hypotension would suggest that both of these entities occur very rarely in the age group under eighteen. Although six cases of jaundice have been reported in the age group one to eighteen, only in one case was the evidence convincing enough for chlorpromazine to be considered the causative agent. Severe hypotension was noted in only one study. Another author, Balridge (152) stated, "Only in hypertensive children (denoting active pathological conditions) does blood pressure seem affected by chlorpromazine."

Some of the drugs in this survey such as the amphetamines and diphenhydramine have been studied over such an extended interval that we can feel comfortable about their safety for children when given in proper dosage. Two others, hydroxyine and deanol, thus far are notable for their mildness and absence of side effects. The minor tranquilizer, meprobamate has apparently induced side effects infrequently in the light of its widespread usage. However dermatitis, purpura, and fever probably on an allergic basis have been reported in adults so that caution must be sustained during its administration.

Drowsiness following too large a dose of the tranquilizers or excessive stimulation in response to more than the proper dosage of a stimulant can always be removed by dose modification. A similar relationship exists between the development of extrapyramidal nervous system manifestations and the phenothiazines or serpasil. Trifluoperazine and fluphenazine are especially likely to produce undesirable central nervous system reactions if the proper titration of dosage is not followed. But all of these reactions are reversible so that awareness by the patient's family and the doctor can be the adequate safeguard. In the latest report of drug-induced extrapyramidal reactions 1472 of 3775 patients (about 200 under the age of nineteen) developed extrapyramidal reactions 23% developed dyskinesia. Children under fifteen had the most severe and most bizarre neuromuscular symptoms. Usually their hyperkinesis was generalized resulting in a clinical picture resembling advanced cases of dystonia musculorum. The older the patient, the more the involvement was restricted to the muscles of neck, face, tongue and upper limbs (9).

Many child psychiatrists are also concerned about possible toxic effects which may have been overlooked because of incomplete hematologic, liver and central nervous system studies (137). These doubts cannot be resolved with statistical data at this time. Our clinical impression based on observations of over 300 children in two out-patient clinics who were given various members of the tranquilizer group, but not given routine continuous laboratory tests, was that no serious irreversible illness appeared during the administration of the drugs. Deleterious effects on personality functioning thus far have been evaluated only with gross criteria.

Definite evidence that a permanent unhealthy personality change resulted from a therapy in which psychopharmaceuticals were used is obviously difficult to establish. We have not seen children who showed persistent manifestations of greater personality disorganization where drugs were the clear cut etiologic factor although we obviously had our quota of treatment failures. We saw no definite evidence that delinquent children were deterred from committing crimes like petty larceny or minor assault. Restlessness or increased irritability following the use of the more potent phenothiazine derivatives did not eventuate in antisocial behavior. Contrariwise, habituation or increased dependency on medication has not been seen.

THE PLACEBO EFFECT

The importance of the doctor-patient relationship and the influence of suggestion in psychiatry tends to maximize the placebo effect. Lasagna and Meier (107) have pointed out that it is a mistaken notion that the placebo merely controls suggestibility. It is also an aid in controlling external factors common to all groups, such as changes in the milieu and spontaneous changes occurring in the course of the disease. We define this placebo effect as one which is independent of or minimally related to the pharmacologic effects of the medication or to the specific effects of the procedure and which operates through a psychological mechanism (148).

Kurland (106) in his excellent review on the placebo states that from a survey of drug studies he found a placebo effect ranging from 4 to 52% always present. In fifteen studies involving 1082 patients, the average significant effectiveness was $35.2\% \pm 2.2\%$ (19). One of these studies (158) concluded that youth was positively related to the placebo response while there was little or no relationship between the response and intelligence, presence of environmental problems or severity of illness. Another study (13) carried out on deteriorated psychotic patients showed highly significant results were obtained with the placebo rather than with phenothiazine. The explanation that the control group responded favorably because they received small sweets daily rather than bitter pills must be considered seriously in dealing with children. We found that a placebo effect was observable in about one-third of all our patients. It was found more often in children who were resistant to attendance in a clinic, in those whose parents were firmly convinced of the value of tranquilizers and in children who were convinced that taking medication meant that they were crazy. Thus we see that a "negative placebo effect" to an underevaluation of a helpful therapeutic effect has to be considered.

Chapter VI

SUMMATION

Is the general practitioner and the child psychiatrist in the clinic justified in exhibiting these potent drugs to growing children whose behavior is no more disturbed than that of the many others who are treated with psychotherapy alone because such treatment is available to them? Freedom versus conformity, all too familiar terms in this world today, are the polar opposites which may pose a problem to the analytically oriented psychiatrists who feel that the use of tranquilizing drugs will take away the child's inalienable right to develop with emotional freedom.

One must agree with the dictum of Hollister (87) that there is no drug yet known which will remove a patient from a stressful environment or influence human behavior and thought as much as persons and ideas do. Furthermore no one has recommended that we should seek a "chemical annihilation of feelings." A team of investigators concerned about the responsibility which goes beyond the present asks what we would be without anxiety, without fear and without guilt (136). It cannot be emphasized too strongly that all of the drugs discussed here are only ameliorative and should be used as adjuncts to some form of psychotherapy.

Dynamic psychotherapy exemplified in the psychoanalytic approach emphasizes watchful waiting and the proper timing of interpretations and interventions. Today dynamic family psychotherapy includes insight gained by the new knowledge garnered from child development and therapy. This combines the analytic attitude of looking backward into the genesis of behavior with the sociological attitude of dealing with the immediate interaction and its current implications. This is also the therapeutic attitude suited to the psychiatrist utilizing psychopharmacologic agents. Frequently he must be a "here and now psychiatrist" (153). That is, he may attempt to expeditiously strengthen the ego by modulating effects or he could seek to promptly diminish that quantity of anxiety which threatens to produce disorganization in the individual and in the family. He is also concerned with the feedback of aggression in the classroom and the subsequent disorganization in the class. Mention must be made of the current thinking in the field of psychotherapy. D. E. Cameron (39) on "The Essence of Psychotherapy" stated, "we should also like to draw attention to the fact that many of our attempts to understand psychotherapeutic processes seem to be based on the assumption that causality is always deterministic. This is by no means the case. We have to take into account that most of the causality at the behavioral level is emergent and, on occasion, seems to be circular." The experiments on sensory deprivation have stimulated Eisenberg (54) to suggest that "if we may reason from a sensory phenomena to the social ones, there is in all this the suggestion that what we see in our patients is less explicable in terms of the past than we have been want to consider. Contemporaneous reinforcement by social cues may account for much of what we take to be intrinsic consistency of personality molded by previous experience." Thus we may be witnessing the convergence of the latest concepts of clinical psychodynamics, neurophysiology and psychopharmacology as we work with the patient—in this case, the child—on the "here and now" aspect of the illness.

We have not been deterred from using a variety of these drugs after gaining some experience with them. We found fewer side effects with these psychopharmaceuticals in children than in adults. None of these effects have been irreversible or even dangerous since we anticipated such a possibility as basal ganglia dysfunction and prepared the parent for such a possibility.

We have used some of these preparations such as chlorpromazine, prochlorperazine, triflupromazine and trifluoperazine (67) in selected cases for periods of one to five years without observing addiction, increased drug tolerance or apparent organ injury during routine observation. We have recognized the personality need to develop tolerance to anxiety and frustration. Follow up observations have not indicated to us that dependency strivings have been fostered nor spontaneity inhibited. It is hoped that continued follow ups may enable us to evaluate such dynamic factors in the personalities of our growing patients. Meanwhile we may find possible clues in animal experimentation with observations on immature organisms. "An interesting experiment on the effects of chlorpromazine upon the psychological development in the puppy" is now available. "The hypothesis that 'tranquilization' lowers the value of experience—that stimuli are less meaningful to a drugged animal and that the organization of adaptive behavior patterns is more or less permanently impaired—was tested. It was predicted that drugged semi-isolated puppies would differ from nondrugged semi-isolated puppies in behavior. In addition drugged and non-drugged subjects were separated into punished and non-punished groups to see if chlorpromazine had differential effects in a generally rewarding situation and one designed to be anxiety producing. The conjecture was that any effects of chlorpromazine would be greater in the punished groups. It was found that the effects of chlorpromazine upon psychological development appeared to be minor or not at all. The experimenters observed, "This may be reassuring to those concerned about the occurrence of learning deficits or other impairments in children chronically treated with chlorpromazine. Yet our failure to demonstrate effects from tranquillization comparable to those of isolation does not mean that drugs cannot modify psychological development. One possibility is that chlorpromazine is a less effective inhibitor of learning than are some other drugs. Hess (1957) for example, has shown that meprobamate interferes with imprinting in ducklings, but chlorpromazine is ineffective" (72).

Undoubtedly psychopharmacological research in children will go on at a slower pace than that in adults. As Uhr and Miller (160) have pointed out, the welfare of children or other groups used as subjects is particularly guarded by the sympathies of the community. Furthermore some thoughtful physicians have strongly questioned the ethics of the use of placebos which are known not to help patients without their consent.

It is likely that we will pursue Wikler's suggestion (162) that we outline patterns of responses to individual drugs rather than isolated reactions to the medication. Figure I may be one possible approach to such a classification.* Rather than selecting a target symptom for treatment, we will, as Fish suggests (59, 60) consider patterns of behavior because of our expanded knowledge of levels of maturation and our increased expectations from the combined approach of a dynamic psychotherapy and a physiologic psychopharmacology.

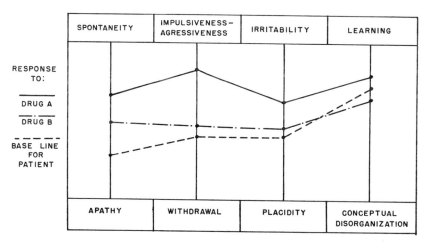

---

*R. Cattell has written extensively of the dimensional measurement of anxiety, effort, stress and other mood reaction patterns. For the irritability-placidity axis he would seem to have a dimension of excitability versus unreactiveness. He has a dimension of mobilization versus debility which might be equated with our axis of aggressiveness versus withdrawal (43).

BIBLIOGRAPHY

1. ADAMSON, W. C., NELLIS, B., RUNGE, G., CLELAND, D., and KIL-
   LIAN, E.: Use of tranquilizers for mentally deficient patients.
   A.M.A.J. Dis. Child., 96:159–164, 1958.
2. A.M.A. COMMITTEE: Personal Communication.
3. ANTON-STEPHENS, D.: Preliminary observations on the psychiatric
   uses of chlorpromazine (Largactil). *J. Ment. Sci. 100*:543–557,
   1954.
4. AYD, F. J. Jr.: Tranquilizing drugs in private practice. *New York
   State J. Med., 57*:1742, May 15, 1957.
5. AYD, F. J. Jr.: Meprobamate therapy for convulsive disorders in
   children. *Bull. School Med. Univ. Maryland, 42*:2, 1957.
6. AYD, F. J. Jr.: Emotional problems in children; use of drugs in
   therapeutic management. *Calif. Med., 87*:2, Aug., 1957.
7. AYD, F. J. Jr.: Drug induced extrapyramidal reactions: Their
   clinical manifestations and treatment with akineton. *Psychoso-
   matics, 1*:1–8, 1960.
8. AYD, F. J. Jr.: Current status of major tranquilizers. *J. Med. Soc.
   N. J., 57*:414, 1960.
9. AYD, F. . Jr.: A survey of drug-induced extrapyramidal reactions.
   J.A.M.A., 175:102–108, 1961.
10. BAIR, H. V. and HEROLD, W.: Efficacy of chlorpromazine in hyper-
    active mentally retarded children. *A.M.A. Arch. Neurol. &
    Psychiat., 74*:363–364, 1955.
11. BAIRD, H. W. III: A comparison of meprospan (sustained action
    meprobamate capsule) with other tranquilizing and relaxing
    agents in children. *J. Pediat., 54*:170, Feb. 1959.
12. BAIRD, H. W. III and BOROFSKY, L. G.: Infantile myoclonic
    seizures. *J. Pediat., 50*:332, 1957.
13. BAKER, A. and THORPE, J.: Placebo response. *Arch. Neurology &
    Psychiatry, 78*:57–60, 1957.
14. BAKWIN, H.: The uses of chlorpromazine in pediatrics. *J. Pediat.,
    48*:240–247, 1956.

15. BARSA, J.A. and KLINE, N. S.: Use of reserpine in disturbed psychotic patients. *Am. J. Psychiat., 112*:684–691, 1956.

16. BATTIATA, S. V. and O'REILLY, W. R.: Untoward reactions following the use of prochlorperazine (Compazine) : A report of two cases. *Clin. Proc. Children's Hosp., 15*:147–150, June, 1959.

17. BAYART, J.: Hydroxyzine in treatment of nervous conditions during childhood. *Acta Paediat. Belg., 10*:164, 1956.

18. BECATTINI, U., and GALLINI, R.: Clinical evaluation of the action of meprobamate, benactyzine and hydroxyzine in the treatment of some psycho-emotional juvenile disorders. In: Garattini, S., and Ghetti, V. (Eds) *Psychotropic Drugs.* Amsterdam, Elsevier Publishing Co. 563–564, 1957.

19. BEECHER, H. K.: The powerful placebo. *J.A.M.A.,* 158, 1602, 1955.

20. BENDA, H: Promazine in mental deficiency *Psych. Quart., 32*:449, 1958.

21. BENDER, L. S.: In: Wolff, W. (Ed) *Contemporary Psychotherapists Examine Themselves.* Thomas, Springfield, 1956.

22. BENDER, L., and COTTINGTON, F.: The use of amphetamine sulfate (Benzedrine) in child psychiatry. *Am. J. Psychiat., 99*:116–121, 1942.

23. BENDER, L. and NICHTERN, S.: Chemotherapy in child psychiatry. *New York State J. Med., 56*:2791, 1956.

24. BERGER, F.: Classification of psychoactive drugs according to their chemical structures and sites of action. In: Uhr, L., and Miller, J. (Eds.) *Drugs and Behavior.* J. Wiley, N. Y. 1960.

25. BERGMAN, P. and ESCALONA, S.: Unusual sensitivities in very young children. Psychoanal. Study of the Child. Vols. *3 & 4*:332–352, 1949.

26. BERMAN, H. J., LAZAR, M. and NOE, O.: Prochlorperazine as an antiemetic in the severely retarded child. *A.M.A. J. Dis. Child., 95*:146–149, 1958.

27. BERMAN, H. J., LAZAR, M., NOE, O. and SCHILLER, H.: Pentylenetetrazol (Metrazol) in mental deficiency. *A.M.A. J. Dis. Child., 94*:231–233, 1957.

28. BINZER, P.: "The Slow Learners"—Philadelphia Evening Bulletin, April 4, 1960.

29. BOWMAN, P., and BLUMBERG, E.: Treatment of hyperactive mentally retarded patients. *Am. J. Ment. Deficiency, 49*:272, 1958.

30. BRADLEY, C.: The behavior of children receiving Benzedrine. *Am. J. Psychiat., 94*:577–585, 1937.

31. BRADLEY, C.: Benzedrine and Dexedrine in the treatment of children's behavior disorders. *Pediatrics, 5*:24–37, 1950.

32. BRADLEY, C.: Tranquilizing drugs in pediatrics. *Pediatrics, 21*:325–326, 1958.

33. BRADLEY, C., and BOWEN, M.: School performance of children receiving amphetamine (Benzedrine) sulphate. *Am. J. Orthopsychiat., 10*:782–788, 1940.

34. BRADLEY, C., and BOWEN, M.: Amphetamine (Benzedrine) therapy in children's behavior disorders. *Am. J. Orthopsychiat., 11*:92–103, 1941.

35. BRADLEY, C. and GREEN, E.: Psychometric performance of children receiving amphetamine (Benzedrine) sulfate. *Am. J. Psychiat., 97*:388–394, 1940.

36. BRADY, J.: Comparative psychopharmacology: Animal experimental studies on the effects of drugs on behavior. In: Cole, J. and Gerard, R. W. (Eds). Psychopharmacology. Washington, D. C. Research Council, 46–63, 1959.

37. BRODIE, B. B.: Comments on a symposium entitled *"A Pharmacologic Approach to the Study of the Mind."* Featherstone, R. and Simon, A. (Eds.) 52–63, Thomas, Springfield, 1959.

38. BRODIE, B. B., OLIN, J., KUNTZMAN, R. G. and SHORE, P.: Possible interrelationship between release of brain norepinephrine and serotonin by reserpine. *Science, 125*:1293–1294, 1957.

39. CAMERON, D. E.: The essence of psychotherapy. Conf. Temple University Medical School. March, 1960.

40. CARES, R. M., ASRICAN, E., FENICHEL, M., SACK, P., and SEVERINO, J.: Therapeutic and toxic effects of chlorpromazine among 3,014 hospitalized cases. *Am. J. Psychiat., 114*:318–327, 1957.

41. CARTER, C. H.: The effect of meprobamate (Equanil) on brain-damaged patients. *Am. J. M. Science, 235*:632, June, 1958.

42. CARTER, H.: Management of behavior disorders in mentally defective children. In: *Trifluoperazine.* Moyer, J. H. (Ed.) 123–129, Lea and Febriger, Phila. 1959.

43. CATTELL, R.: The dimensional (unitary component) measurement of anxiety, excitement, effort, stress and other mood reaction patterns. In: Uhr, L. and Miller, J. (Eds.) *Drugs and Behavior,* J. Wiley, N.Y., 438–462, 1960.

44. CHRISTIAN, C. D. and PAULSON, G.: Severe motility disturbances after small doses of prochlorperazine. *New England J. Med., 239*:828–839, Oct. 1958.

45. CLAUSEN, J., FINEMAN, M., HENRY, C. and WHOL, N.: The effect of Deaner on mentally retarded subjects. *Training School Bulletin (Vineland, N. J.)*, 57:3–12, 1960.

46. CLEVELAND, W. W. and SMITH, G. F.: Complications following the use of prochlorperazine "Compazine" as an anti-emetic. *A.M.A. J. Dis. Child., 96*:284–287, Sept. 1958.

47. COLE, J. O.: Drug Therapy. In: Spiegel, E. A. (Ed.) *Progress in Neurology and Psychiatry* (Vol. XV, 1960,) Grune & Stratton, N. Y.

48. CRAFT, M.: Tranquilizers in mental deficiency: Hydroxyzine. *J. Ment. Sci., 103*:855–857, 1957.

49. CUTLER, M., LITTLE, J. W., and STRAUSS, A. A.: Effect of Benzedrine on mentally deficient children. *Am. J. Ment. Deficiency., 45*:59–65, 1960.

50. CYTRYN, L., GILBERT, S. and EISENBERG, L.: The effectiveness of tranquilizing drugs plus supportive psychotherapy in behavior disorders of children. Double blind study of 80 out-patients. *Am. J. Orthopsychiatry, 30*:113–129, 1960.

51. DARYN, E.: Problem of children with "diffuse brain damage." Archives of Gen. *Psychiatry, 4*:299–306, 1961.

52. DiMASCIO, J., and KLERMAN, G.: Experimental human psychopharmacologic role of non-drug factors. In: Sarwer-Foner, G. (Ed.) *The Dynamics of Psychiatric Therapy.* 56–78, Thomas, Springfield, 1960.

53. EHRMANTRAUT, W. R., NEGRON, M. D., KLEH, J. and FAZEKAS, J. F.: Effects of combination of psychopharmacologic agents. *Am. J. Science, 238*:412, 1959.

54. EISENBERG, S.: Conceptual problems in relating brain and behavior, *Am. J. Orthopsychiatry, 30*:37–48, 1960.

55. ESCALONA, S.: The impact of psychoanalysis upon child psychology. *J. Nerv. & Mental Diseases, 126*:429–441, 1958.

56. ESEN, F. M. and DURLING, D.: The treatment of 14 mentally retarded boys with Sparine. *Arch. Pediat., 74*:471–474, 1957.

57. ESEN, F. M., and DURLING, D.: Thorazine in the treatment of mentally retarded children. *Arch. Pediat., 73*:168–173, 1956.

58. FABIAN, A. A.: Reading disability: an index of pathology. *Am. J. Orthopsychiatry, 25:*319–330, 1955.

59. FISH, B.: Drug therapy in child psychiatry—psychologic aspects, *Comprehensive Psychiatry, 1:*55–61, 1960.

60. FISH, B.: Drug therapy in child psychiatry—pharmacological aspects. *Comprehensive Psychiatry, 1:*212–227, 1960.

61a. FISHER, E.: Reserpine (Serpasil) in mental deficiency practice. *J. Ment. Sci., 102:*542–545, 1956.

61b. FISHER, S., (ED.): *Child Research in Psychophormacology.* Springfield, Thomas, 1959.

62. FLAHERTY, J. A.: Effect of chlorpromazine medication on children with severe emotional disturbance. *Delaware State Med. J., 27:*180–184, 1955.

63. FREED, H.: On the parenteral use of amitriptyline (Elavil-Merck). A preliminary report. *Am. J. Psychiatry.,* Vol. 117, No. 5, Nov. 1960.

64. FREED, H.: Some preliminary observations on the use of Vesprin in children and adults. *Monogr. Ther., 2:*197–202, 1957.

65. FREED, H.: The tranquilizing drugs and the school child. *American Practitioner, 8:*377–380, 1957.

66. FREED, H.: On special uses of diphenhydramine hydrochloride in the somatic therapy ward of a psychiatric hospital. *Am. J. Psychiatry, 115:*359, 1958.

67. FREED, H., and FRIGNITO, N.: Current status of the tranquilizers in child psychiatry with particular reference to the phenothiazines. (Presented at Pan American Medical Congress, May 4, 1960, Mexico City). In Press.

68. FREED, H., and PEIFER, C. A.: Treatment of hyperkinetic emotionally disturbed children with prolonged administration of chlorpromazine. *Am. J. Psychiatry, 113:*22–26, 1956.

69. FREED, H., ABRAMS, J. and PEIFER, C. A.: Reading disability: a new therapeutic approach and its implications. *J. Clin. and Experimental Psychopathology, 20:* No. 3. July-Sept. 1959.

70. FREEDMAN, A. M.: Drug therapy in behavior disorders. *Pediatric Clin. North America, 5:*573–584, 1958.

71. FREEDMAN, A. M., KREMER, M. W., ROBERTIELLO, R. C. and EFFRON, A. S.: The treatment of behavior disorders in children with Tolserol. *J. Pediat., 47:*369–372, 1955.

72. FULLER, J. L., CLARK, L. D. and WALLER, M. B.: Effects of chlor-

promazine upon the psychological development in the puppy. *Psychopharmacologia, 1*:393–407, 1960.

73. GATSKI, R. L.: Chlorpromazine in the treatment of emotionally maladjusted children. *J.A.M.A., 157*:1298–1300, 1955.

74. GELLER, S.: Comparison of a tranquilizer and psychic energizer. *J.A.M.A., 174*:481–484, 1960.

75. GEVER, H. W.: Response to Thorazine (chlorpromazine) administration in hyperkinetic mongolism. *Delaware State Med. J., 28*:189–190, 1956.

76. GOLDSMITH, R. W.: Antidote for prochlorperazine intoxication in children. *J.A.M.A., 170*–361, May 16, 1959.

77. HERSCHEL, P.: The tranquilizing drugs: Unfavorable effects in children. *Kaiser Foundation Med. Bulletin, 7*:61–73, April-June, 1959.

78. HESS, W. R.: Diencephalon: autonomic and extrapyramidal functions. Vol. III. *Monographs in Biology & Medicine.* N. Y. Grune & Stratton.

79. HESS, E. H.: Effects of meprobamate on imprinting in water fowl. *Ann. New York Acad. Sci., 67*:724–733, 1957.

80. HEUYER, G., LANG, J. L. and CHEVREAU, J. P.: First results of a chlorbenzhydral derivative in child psychiatry. *Encephale, 45*:579, 1956.

81. HILL, D.: Amphetamine in psychopathic states. *Brit. J. Addiction, 44*:50–54, 1947.

82. HIMWICH, H.: Tranquilizers, barbiturates and the brain. Exhibit A.P.A. Atlantic City, N. J., May, 1960.

83. HIMWICH, H., COSTA, E., RINALDI, F., and RUDY, L.: Trifluoromazine and trifluoperazine in the treatment of disturbed mentally defective patients. *Am. J. Ment. Deficiency, 64*:711–712, 1960.

84. HOCH, P.: Drugs and psychotherapy. *Am. J. Psycho., 116*:305–308, 1959.

85. HOFFER, A.: Discussion, *Canada Psycho. Assoc. Journal, 4*:5119, 1959 (special supplement).

86. HODGE, R. S. and HUTCHINGS, H. M.: Enuresis: A brief review; a tentative theory and a suggested treatment. *Arch. Dis. Child. 27*:498–504, 1952.

87. HOLLISTER, L. E.: Drugs in emotional disorders: Past and present. *Ann. Int. Medicine, 51*:1032–1048, 1959.

88. HOLLISTER, L. E.: Allergic reactions to tranquilizing drugs. *Ann. of Int. Medicine, 49*:17. July, 1958.

89. HOLLISTER, L. E. and GLAZNER, F. S.: Withdrawal reaction to meprobamate alone and combined with promazine. Psychopharmacologia. In Press.

90. HUGHES, J. C. and JABBOUR, J. T.: The treatment of the epileptic child. *J. Pediat., 53*:66, 1958.

91. HUNT, B., FRANK, T. and KRUSH, T.: Chlorpromazine in the treatment of severe emotional disorders of children. *A.M.A. J. Dis. Child., 91*:268, 1956.

92. HUXLEY, J.: Discussion. *Ann. New York Acad. Sci., 67*:732, 1957.

93. IRWIN, S.: Use of drugs to modify the social behavior of animals. In: Denber, H. (Ed.): *Therapeutic Community*. Thomas, Springfield, 1960.

94. IRWIN, S.: The value of animal experimentation. In: Kline, N. (Ed.) *Psychopharmacology Frontiers*. Little, Brown & Co. Boston, 1959.

95. ISON, M. G.: Effect of Thorazine on Wechsler Score. *Am. J. Ment. Deficiency, 64*:57–62, 1959.

96. JABBOUR, J. T., SHEFFIELD, J. and MONTALVO, J.: Severe neurological manifestations in four children receiving "Compazine" (prochlorperazine). *J. Pediat., 53* (2):153–159., Aug. 1958.

97. KATZ, B. E.: Education of cerebral palsied children—The role of meprobamate: A preliminary evaluation. *J. Pediat., 53*:467, 1958.

98. KLEH, J., EHRMANTRAUT, W. and FAZEKAS, J. F.: The choice of psychotrophic drugs in the treatment of neuropsychiatric disorders. In: Garattini, S. and Ghetti, V. (Eds.) *Psychotrophic Drugs*. Elsevier, Amsterdam. 515–526, 1957.

99. KLINE, N.: Psychopharmaceuticals—effects and side effects. *Bulletin of World Health Organization, 21*:397–410, 1959.

100. KLINE, N.: Neusopsychiatric disorders. In: Waife, S. and Shapiro, A. (Eds.) *Clinical Evaluation of Drugs*. 195–213, Hoeber and Harper, N. Y. 1959.

101. KLINE, N. (Ed.): *Psychopharmacology Frontiers*. Little, Brown and Co. Boston, 1959.

102. KNOBEL, M., WOLMAN, M. and MASON, E.: Hyperkinesis and organicity in children. *A.M.A. Archives of Gen. Psych., 1*:310–321, 1959.

103. Kovitz, B.: Management of psychotic tension symptoms with Trifluoperazine: A preliminary report. In: *Trifluoperazine: Clinical and Pharmacological Aspects.* Lea & Febiger. Phila. 1958.

104. Kraft, I. A., Marcus, I. M., Wilson, W., Swander, D., Rummage, N. and Schulhofer, E.: Methodological problems in studying effects of tranquilizers in children with special reference to meprobamate. *Southern Med. Assoc. Miami Beach,* Nov. 11-14, 1957. Also *South M. J. 52:*179, 1959.

105. Kugelmass, I. N.: Psychochemotherapy of mental deficiency in children. *Internat. Record of Medicine and General Practice Clinics. 169:*323–338, 1956.

106. Kurland, A.: Placebo effect. In: Uhr, L. and Miller, J. (Eds.) *Drugs and Behavior.* J. Wiley, N. Y. 1960.

107. Lasagna, L. and Meier, P.: In: Waife, S. and Shapiro, A. (Eds.) *Clinical Evaluation of New Drugs.* 37-60. Hoeber and Harper, N. Y. 1959.

108. Laufer, M. W., Denhoff, E. and Solomon, C.: Hyperkinetic impulse disorder in children's behavior problems. *Psychosomatic Med., 19:*38–39, 1957.

109. Laufer, M. W., Denhoff, E. and Rubin, E.: Photo-metrazol activation in children. *EEG Clin. Neurophys., 6:*1–8, 1954.

110. LaVann, L.: The use of trifluoperazine as a tranquilizing agent in mentally defective children. In: *Trifluoperazines Clinical and Pharmacological Aspects.* Lea & Febiger. Phila. 1959.

111. Lehman, H.: Haber, J. and Lesser, S. F.: The effects of reserpine in autistic children. *J. Nerv & Ment. Dis., 126:*351–356, 1957.

112. Lehmann, H.: Concepts, rationale and research. In: Kline, N. (Ed.) *Psychopharmacology Frontiers.* Little, Brown & Co. Boston, 1959.

113. Lehmann, H. E., and Knight, D. A.: Psychophysiologic testing with a new phrenotrophic drug. In: *Trifluoperazines Clinical and Pharmacological Aspects.* Lea & Febiger. Phila. 1959.

114. Lilly, J. C.: The psychophysiological basis for two kinds of instincts. *J. Am. Psychoanalytic A., 8:*659–670, Oct. 1960.

115. Litchfield, H. R.: Clinical pediatric experience with ataractic agent in less severe emotional states. *New York State J. of Med.,* Vol. 60, No. 4, Feb. 15, 1960.

116. Litchfield, H. R.: Clinical evaluation of meprobamate in dis-

turbed and prepsychotic children. *Ann. New York Acad. Sci.,* 67:828, May 9, 1957.

117. LIVINGSTON, S. and PAULI, L.: Meprobamate in the treatment of epilepsy of children. *A.M.A. J. Dis. Child., 84*:277, 1957.

118. MacDONALD, R. and WATTS, T. P.: Trifluoperazine dihydrochloride "Stelazine" in paranoid schizophrenia. *Brit. Med. J., 1*:549–550, Feb. 28, 1959.

119. MAHLER, M., FURER, M. & SETTLAGE, C.: Severe emotional disturbances in childhood. In: *American Handbook of Psychiatry.* Vol. 1:816–839, Basic Books, N. Y. 1959.

120. MASON, S. R., SANDT, J., and DUGGAN, J.: Acute, transitory, severe central nervous system toxicity following administration of prochlorperazine. *New York State J. Med., 59*:2037–40, 1959.

121. MASSERMAN, J.: *Dynamic Psychiatry,* Saunders, Phila. 1955.

122. McCLENDON, S. J.: Management of nocturnal enuresis in childhood. *Arch. Pediat., 75*:101, March, 1958.

123. MIKSZTAL, M. W.: Chlorpromazine (Thorazine) and reserpine in residental treatment of neuro-psychiatric disorders. *J. Nerv. & Ment. Diseases, 125*:477, 1956.

124. MITCHELL, A., HARGIS, C., McCARREY, F., and POWERS, C.: Effects of prochlorperazine (Compazine) treatment on educability of disturbed mentally retarded adolescents. *Am. J. Ment. Deficiency, 64*:57–62, 1959.

125. OETTINGER, L.: The use of deanol in the treatment of disorders of behavior in children. *J. Pediat., 53*:671–675, 1958.

126. OETTINGER, L.: Personal Communication.

127. O'HARA, U. S.: Extrapyramidal reactions in patients receiving prochlorperazine. *New England J. Med., 239*:826–828, Oct. 1958.

128. OSTOW, N. and KLINE, N.: Psychic action of resperine and chlorpromazine. In: Kline, N. (Ed.) *Psychopharmacology Frontiers.* 481–513. Little, Brown & Co. Boston. 1959.

129. OUNSTED, C.: The hyperkinetic syndrome in epileptic children. *Lancet, 2*:303–311, 1955.

130. PALLESTER, D., and STEVENS, R.: Effects of serpasil in small dosage on behavior, intelligence and psychiology. *Am. J. Ment. Deficiency. 63*:330, 1958.

131. PALMER, E. and WRIGHT, C.: Some experiences with the use of Deaner in retarded children. Presented at annual meeting of Nat. Assoc. for Retarded Children. Phila. Oct. 8, 1958.

132. PAUIG, P., DELUCA, M. and OSTERHELD, R.: Thioridazine HCl in treatment of behavior disorders in epileptics. *Am. J. Psych., 117:* 832–833, 1961.

133. PEARSON, H. J.: Psychoanalysis and the education of the child. W. W. North, N. Y. 1954.

134. PERLSTEIN, M. A.: Use of meprobamate (Miltown) in convulsive and related disorders. *J.A.M.A., 161:* 1040, July 14, 1956.

135. PERLSTEIN, M. A.: The use of a monamine oxidase inhibitor (Catron) in behavior disturbances in children. In: Featherstone, R. and Simon, A. (Eds.) *Pharmacologic Study of the Mind.* 362–370. Thomas, Springfield, 1959.

136. POLLARD, J. and BAKKER, C.: Drugs and Behavior. Uhr, L. and Miller, J. (Eds) 198–208. J. Wiley, N. Y. 1960.

137. PRUGH, D.: Personal Communication.

138. RAWITT, K.: The usefulness and effectiveness of Equanil in children. *Am. J. Psych., 115:* 1120–1121, 1959.

139. RETTIG, J. H.: Chlorpromazine for the control of psychomotor excitement in the mentally deficient: A preliminary study. *J. Nerv. and Ment. Dis., 122:* 190–194, 1955.

140. ROCHLIN, G.: The loss complex. *J.A.P.A., 7:* 298–316, 1959.

141. ROSENBLUM, S., CALLAHAN, R. J., BUONICONTO, P., GRAHAM, B., and DEATRICK, R. W.: The effects of tranquilizing medication (Reserpine) on behavior and test performance of maladjusted, high-grade retarded children. *Am. J. Ment. Deficiency, 62:* 663–671, 1958.

142. ROSENBLUM, S., and BUONICONTO, P.: "Compazine" vs. placebo: A controlled study with educable emotionally disturbed children. *Am. J. Ment. Deficiency, 64:* 713–717, 1960.

143. SAUNDERS, J. C.: Phenelzine in childhood and adolescent psychiatric disturbances. Paper presented before section in Child Psychiatry, Pan American Medical Congress, May 4, 1960.

144. SAUNDERS, J., RICHLIN, D., RADINGER, N. and KLINE, N.: Iproniazid in depressed and regressed patients. In: Kline, N. (Ed.) *Psychopharmacology Frontiers,* 177–194. Little, Brown & Co. Boston, 1959.

145. SAVAGE, A.: Transference and countertransference as aspect of tranquilizing drugs. In: Sarwer-Foner, G. (Ed.) *The Dynamics of Psychiatric Therapy,* 369–375. Thomas, Springfield, 1960.

146. SCHIELE, B. C. and BENSON, W.: Tranquilizing and related drugs;

a guide for the general physician. *Post. Grad. Med., 23*:484, 1958.

147. SCIME, I. A. and TALLANT, E. J.: Tetanus-like reactions to prochlorperazine (Compazine). *J.A.M.A., 171*:1813–1817, Nov. 28, 1959.

148. SHAPIRA, A.: The placebo effect in the history of medical treatment: implications for psychiatry. *Am. J. Psych., 116*:298–304, 1959.

149. SHAW, E. B.: Convulsive seizures following phenothiazine tranquilizers. *Pediatrics, 22*:175–176, July, 1958.

150. SKINNER, B.: *Science and Human Behavior.* Macmillan, 1955.

151. SOLLEY, C. and MURPHY, C.: *Development of the Perceptual World.* Basic Books, N. Y. 1960.

152. SMITH, KLINE and FRENCH: Personal Communication.

153. STEIGER, WM.: Personal Communication.

154. STRAUSS, A. A. and LEHTINEN, L. E.: *Psychopathology and Education of the Brain Injured Child.* Vol. 1, Grune & Stratton, N. Y. 1957.

155. SZASZ, T.: Some observations on the use of tranquilizing drugs. *A.M.A. Archives of Neurol. & Psych., 77*:86–92, 1957.

156. TARJAN, G.: Research in mental deficiency with emphasis on etiology. *Bull. of Menninger Clinic, 24*:57–69, 1960.

157. TARJAN, G., LOWERY, V. E. and WRIGHT, S. W.: Use of chloropromazine in two hundred seventy-eight mentally deficient patients. *A.M.A. J. Dis. Child., 94*:294–300, 1957.

158. TIBBETS, R. W. and HAWKINS, J. R.: The placebo response. *J. Ment. Science, 102*:60–66, 1956.

159. TIMBERLAKE, W. H., BELMONT, E. H., and OGONIK, J.: The effect of reserpine in two hundred mentally retarded children. *Am. J. Ment. Deficiency, 62*:61–66, 1957.

160. UHR, L., and MILLER, J. (Eds.): *Drugs and Behavior.* J. Wiley, N. Y. 1960.

161. WARDELL, D., RUBIN, H., and ROSS, R.: Use of reserpine and chlorpromazine in disturbed mentally defective patients. *Am. J. Ment. Deficiency, 63*:330, 1958.

162. WIKLER, A.: Some problems in experimental psychiatry. Psychiatrics Research Reports #9. 89–112, 1958.

163. ZARLING, V. and HOGAN, J.: Control of the organic hyperkinetic behavior syndrome in the elementary school child. Scientific

Exhibit, American Academy of Pediatrics, Chicago, Act. 5-8, 1959.

164. ZIMMERMAN, F. T. and BURGMEISTER, B. B.: Effects of reserpine on the behavior problems of children. *New York State J. Med.*, *57*:3132–3140, 1957.

INDEX